Because Trauma…

Because Trauma…

By: Sally Taylor

Sally Taylor

Table of Contents:

Dedication –	Page 4
Note From Author –	Page 5
Chapter One –	Page 12
Chapter Two –	Page 17
Chapter Three –	Page 21
Chapter Four –	Page 25
Chapter Five –	Page 31
Chapter Six –	Page 36
Chapter Seven –	Page 42
Chapter Eight –	Page 47
Chapter Nine –	Page 50
Chapter Ten –	Page 53
Chapter Eleven –	Page 59
Chapter Twelve –	Page 63
Chapter Thirteen –	Page 65
Chapter Fourteen –	Page 70
Chapter Fifteen –	Page 75
Chapter Sixteen –	Page 79
Chapter Seventeen –	Page 84
Chapter Eighteen –	Page 88
Chapter Nineteen –	Page 92
Chapter Twenty –	Page 96
Chapter Twenty-One –	Page 101
Chapter Twenty-Two –	Page 106
Chapter Twenty-Three –	Page 111
Chapter Twenty-Four –	Page 115
Chapter Twenty-Five –	Page 121
Chapter Twenty-Six –	Page 125
Chapter Twenty-Seven –	Page 128

Chapter Twenty-Eight –	Page 133
Chapter Twenty-Nine –	Page 136
Chapter Thirty –	Page 141
Chapter Thirty-One –	Page 146
Chapter Thirty-Two –	Page 148
Chapter Thirty-Three –	Page 153
Chapter Thirty-Four –	Page 156
Chapter Thirty-Five –	Page 162
Chapter Thirty-Six –	Page 166
Chapter Thirty-Seven –	Page 170
Chapter Thirty-Eight –	Page 175
Chapter Thirty-Nine –	Page 180
Chapter Forty –	Page 185
Chapter Forty-One –	Page 189
Reflection –	Page 192
Chapter Forty-Two –	Page 193
Chapter Forty-Three –	Page 199
Chapter Forty-Four –	Page 206
Chapter Forty-Five –	Page 211
Because Trauma (Poetry) –	Page 217
References –	Page 222
Final Thoughts –	Page 225
End –	Page 226

Sally Taylor

Because Trauma…

Sally Taylor

I dedicate this book in memory of my grandmother. Her faith and belief in God, and other people was unwavering. It was something I greatly admired about her.

Because Trauma…

Note from the author:

I understand that this information may not resonate with everyone. I also know I've not experienced the worst traumatic experiences and many people have been through so much worse. My hopes are that this book provides understanding or help to someone that needs it. I'm not trying to impress the world about things I've overcome, I really didn't expect I would ever write anything like this. I actually didn't see the value in writing this until over a year after I started writing it. During that time, I was in a very dark place mentally and had to really make some difficult decisions on where I was going in life. Through many mistakes, I prevailed and pushed myself to get on track with a plan at a better future. With all this being said, it took me over 20 years to admit to anything in this book and actually begin to open up and let people in my view point. I do not want people to be led to the understanding that I am a mentally strong person, the fact that it took over 20 years for any of this information to be known about me proves I'm not.

Staying quiet for so many years, not letting anyone in is not a strong person. This idea of a book only sparked thanks to my psychiatrist and therapist. In 2019 I was diving deep into my darkness to find the answers I was most afraid of. That led to me finally finding my truths to why it was so difficult for me to let anyone in, including my therapist and psychiatrist. I started jotting down thoughts of why I kept so much secret and why I felt I was unable to communicate what was really going on. It was two weeks that I seriously thought I wouldn't make it and would end up committing suicide. I survived the two weeks and got half a notebook full of answers that resonated with me. I first read about two pages to my therapist. It's all the session had time for. My mind during the session was on full panic. But at the end of the session, I felt so numb and I didn't really know what to feel. Before I left, I asked my therapist if it would be smart to let my psychiatrist know of the notebook. I already knew the answer was yes but I was hoping somehow, I would be wrong. My therapist responded with a strong recommendation that I show my psychiatrist. The next psychiatrist appointment I brought the notebook with me.

Instead of me reading the first two pages to my psychiatrist like I did with my therapist, I just handed the notebook to my psychiatrist letting him take control of what he read and of how much. I sat there in complete panic for what seemed like ages but was really only a few minutes, as he read through each point quickly to get through the entire content. He made a few comments as he read to show me that he understood what he was reading. It was helpful that he did that because I've accepted years ago that no one is truly capable of understanding. This was the first appointment where I truly felt heard and understood.

I did not expect the comment after he read through all the content and I have to accept that it freaked me out a lot. I take his comment as a complement but the process to get the complement was a challenge. He said that the notebook was "the holy grail" of information that medical professionals could ever get to understand people that have been through trauma. I'm not proud to admit it took a bit of trauma from myself to drag up all the answers and details in the book. It took two weeks of being hit with flashback after flashback. It took the close moments where I wanted to give up and just end my existence because it would be so much less painful. After I finished the notebook, I could barely look at it because I had such hatred towards the content. But after hearing the comment from my psychiatrist of it being "the holy grail" of information, I forced myself not to destroy the notebook. Around this time, when I was finding answers and digging up truths that I would rather leave hidden, I was attending college. I was taking three classes. So, I was struggling to find a balance between studying, homework, classes, and personal life. I made a promise to myself at the start of going back to school. I established a line that I wasn't supposed to cross, to not include any personal family drama in the classes. I was to go to school and simply focus on my time there. I learned quickly into the first year of attending classes that I'd have to break that promise. My first poetry class for my Creative Writing minor threw a wrench into my plans, in order to pass the class; I had to include real emotion of real personal situations I've dealt with from my past or current. I tried to just appeal to a general emotion starting out but was called out by my professor to include something real from my experiences. The promises I made was to not drag any personal or family topics into either class. School was going to be my escape to some normalcy. I had failed because one of my classes needed real content, real emotion to be able to succeed in the class. I had to drag some real personal stuff into the class. Thus, the start of really letting people in my views and giving people a chance to understand me better.

Time kept going and life continued and when it got very late in the semester, about 6 class days left to attend, roughly a month; I noticed that the notebook that I hated that my psychiatrist gave such an incredible complement on was still processing in the back of my mind, this being almost a month after I gave him the notebook. One Monday morning I decided that I was not done with the notebook. I decided to not only expand on content but get more personal and real about it. I decided to write a book on the content. My hopes are it helps someone that is going through such a tough time and is in need of help. If anything, my hope is it could help medical professionals understand the mind of someone who has been through trauma a little better. But if I fail on both of those hopes, then I hope it is a way to help myself, a way to process, maybe find answers; and close a chapter in my life to move on to better things.

And that's where the book idea stayed for many months, with not much progress and very little regard for how great it could be. I questioned even continuing this book, asking so many times why anyone would care enough to read this. Why my view of traumatic experiences even mattered? Who would actually go out of their way to buy and read this? I failed to see the value because I still was sorting through most the darker traumatic moments, and I was afraid because I knew that writing this book meant really diving deep into all my traumatic past experiences to really process through and find a way to heal. And that was the worst-case scenario for me then, because I had been trying to outrun my past for so many years and was afraid it would now be too much to handle.

It was a difficult decision, but I eventually started to see the value in this book and became more motivated to get it done. There really is something to the motivation, drive and excitement to completing a project, because that has the amazing power to overcome the greatest fear. And that's how it all really took off with this book, I finally saw the potential and how important it was to complete and little by little I wrote.

I know this content will not resonate with everyone, I hope something will be relatable and understandable. There are points in this book that I can explain well based on my own experiences, but I know that my experiences are not it, other people have different answers and different view-points that resonate better. I have done some research to try to find all possible reasons for a wide range of answers but there may be some that I miss. I'm not perfect, I don't strive to be, I just strive to do my best. Because I have it stuck in my mind that perfection doesn't exist and it's more of a myth than truth.

So, I can't promise perfection, but I can promise that I will do an insane amount of research to gather a great deal of information and work it all into a book that can be read and hopefully understood. I don't expect someone to start reading from page one and continue to the last page in one read. I recommend that it not be done. Because I know that this information can be triggering to some people, I know it can possibly spark flashbacks for some. If anyone reading this find it difficult to get though, I ask to step away for a bit to recover and I also ask, why you are reading it and if maybe it's not the right time for you, the reader, to dive into this content. I give anyone reading this book permission to stop, throw away the book or burn it; if it's too much and you're mentally struggling. Do what you need to feel better, stop reading and destroy the book if you need to, or wait until you've gotten to that mindset where you can read it. The worst outcome for me on this book would be to spark more traumatic experiences or thoughts from a reader and the reader acts in harming themselves or someone else. That is not the goal of this book. The goal is to give information to help. Harm defeats that goal and actually does the opposite. I'm going to try to be as real as I can with my experiences in this book. I know it will be challenging in some moments where I would become vague. It's actually a great defense I have to protect myself that more often than not, I'm not aware of when I start to be vague. It's an unconscious defensive trait for me at the moment. I will do my best to be as real, as detailed, and as informative as I can and try to limit the vagueness to a bare minimum. I'll also have to read through my work and be critical in asking if something's too vague, to try to rewrite what is. With that being said, I know you didn't buy this book to read about my ranting, on with the main content of this book. Thanks for sticking with me this far…

Because Trauma…

Chapter One

My Thoughts: How do I define trauma?

In my experience, I've noticed that trauma varies from person to person. Though everyone can experience trauma, not one trauma is traumatic for everyone. Thinking back to my childhood, there have been a string of minor car accidents that my family have been in, the majority of which are so minor that no one is hurt but vehicles need to be repaired. Many of these accidents are from deer running right into the side of our old Chrysler Sebring Convertible. My step-brother drove the Sebring as he was learning to drive with his permit and had been driving during each deer attack in a matter of 18 months. Then, in 2017 he was in another accident that he couldn't shake off and to this day is still traumatized by it. I've been in just as many fender-benders and accidents as my step-brother and I'm still loving the freedom of driving; but my step-brother is terrified of driving at night and still uneasy to drive in general. For him, car accidents are his traumatic experiences; and though I've been through just as many, I'm fine with getting in my car and just driving.

Because Trauma...

Car accidents are considered to be a possible trauma or lead to someone having difficulty with Post-Traumatic Stress Disorder. But not everyone who gets in car accidents will develop problems with trauma. I tend to go out late at night just to drive because I like it, it's therapeutic for me. But where I'm not hindered by trauma whereas my step-brother is, there are other things where I do struggle and my step-brother shakes it off like nothing.

My step-brother and I have dealt with our parent's divorce in very different ways. My step-brother understands that he's developed an anxiety disorder and regularly takes anxiety medication to combat that, though I deal with anxiety just like him I have a different problem that I've developed from our parent's divorce. Something, my step-brother, can't relate to. I closed myself off from people. I refuse to allow myself to date or fall in love and find my forever person to be with because I'm afraid it won't work out and I can't handle the hurt when it doesn't. I'd rather not even try and not be hurt by it rather than allow myself to be in a dating relationship and fall in love. I don't let anyone close to me. If someone starts to get close, I panic and destroy the relationship. I usually flee, cut ties, run, and disappear.

My step-brother deals with an anxiety disorder that he manages even though it's quite challenging. But he found someone to fall in love with and has started a life with this person, he didn't take the path of shutting everyone out and actually let someone in. Both of us have been traumatized by our parent's divorce. It wasn't the easiest divorce, my parents said they wanted to make it easy for my step-brother and me but then got carried away with dragging us into the ugliness. Sure, my dad left the house to my mom, step-brother and I but, when they'd try pinning us against each other as if trying to convince us to take sides; that's where the real damage happened to my step-brother and me.

I'm a people pleaser. It's not a great thing to be because you get taken advantage of. I'm working on it, and have made so much progress; but at the time of my parents' divorce, I just wanted to make peace between everyone. When both parents were saying horrible and even hateful things about each other trying to convince me and my step-brother to take their side, it's a nasty game of tug-of-war with my emotions that I still don't believe I've recovered from. I believe it's why I refuse to let myself get close to anyone and find someone I can spend the rest of my life with.

It's not just car accidents and divorce between parents that makes for traumatic experiences. There's also death of a loved one or someone close, natural disaster, abuse, violence, witnessing a violent act or murder, rape, and many other situations that can be very traumatic for some; but something that other's may be able to deal with and get over naturally. That's not to say that anyone is better because no one is immune to trauma, it just depends on the situation and the individual's past experiences tied in with what they are equipped to deal with.

Dealing with trauma is a different story. I know I haven't taken the best approach to managing after a traumatic event. I still refuse to fall in love, so even being aware of this and knowing it's not logical; I still can't bring myself to date or give anyone a chance. Aside from my lack of relationship story, there's many emotional responses like outbursts and flashbacks, depression and anxiety, anger and irritability, grief and hopelessness; trauma knows no bounds to emotions. Along with emotional responses there can be physical responses, like sleep disturbances of either too much or too little, eating too much or too little, headaches and many other physical symptoms.

I see trauma as a personalized situation that some people have difficulty dealing with whereas others don't have as much trouble and vice-versa. Trauma is your own body and mind in an extreme panic and survival mode, too stressed to know what to do so you spark the fight, flight or flee response without even appropriately knowing how to deal with the emotional fallout during or afterwards. I see trauma as something you later find as a tool for strength, but it may take years battling with those demons before finding it as a tool. I see trauma as a situation where someone didn't understand or value the needs of another enough to know they were being traumatized. I see trauma as a life changer, but only if you give it that power; don't let trauma defeat but be the driving force for change. Learn from it, improve yourself, get to something better, be better. Even with all that, trauma is a problem that shouldn't be. It is, and it's unfortunate; I'm sorry for anyone dealing with their own traumas, but know that you are not alone and everyone is capable of going through traumatic events and struggling with them. That doesn't lessen your trauma or have the understanding of you being weak. My hope, is that it brings piece of mind knowing that you are not alone. You don't have to deal with it alone.

    Trauma becomes a problem when it negatively affects you daily life. If you start to avoid certain situations because you're afraid that you'd end up in a similar situation as a previous traumatic situation, you've got a problem. If you're isolating yourself and shutting out everyone who loves and cares for you, it's a problem. If you're going through flashbacks, nightmares and situations where it feels like you're reliving the traumatic event even when you're not, it could be Post-Traumatic Stress Disorder and it's a problem. It takes finding the courage to allow someone to help if they are trying or finding it in yourself to be able to ask for help. It's not easy, and there are so many reasons or excuses you'd tell yourself to justify not finding help.

Because Trauma…

Chapter Two

Heart beating faster, now

pain ruling your fear, now

Response: "I don't understand..."

A common thing many people struggle with is admitting that they don't know or don't understand. With the pressures of people expecting relevant answers to questions there a fear or almost a subtle panic when someone doesn't know to find an answer, and the one they found, sounds right but they struggle to confirm it as truth. There are a good number of people that do understand that just being real and responding with "I don't know," or "I don't understand myself," is a very acceptable answer and is more respected than giving an answer that sounds good. By responding with I don't know or don't understand, you show the person seeking an answer that you are not trying to show people that you are perfect and have all the answers and you are in fact, only human.

It intimidates people when someone tries to show that they are so perfect, maybe even better, than others and it's a trait that can lead to distrust. Showing that you are human, and being genuine and real with people can help in building trust and respect. You don't have to know everything. No one in this world does. Everyone has their own collected knowledge on things and everyone brings their own edge or creative ideas to the table. It involves accepting that diversity exists and everyone is valued as an individual, it's a key tool in life. It is not an easy thing to master and can take years to a lifetime to really accomplish it.

But with practice and patience, improvements will happen. Don't doubt yourself from the start and lead yourself to think you are incapable of this. It's a skill anyone can master because you are human. Accept that you will make mistakes. Because you will, you just have to acknowledge that mistake and figure out a different way to not make the same mistake again. That's where you grow and learn. Without the mistakes, you can't grow or learn. There will be no improvement. I'm not saying be proud of the mistakes, just acknowledge that there are mistakes and use them as a learning tool.

For me, I make many mistakes. Many of them I am not proud of. Many I have a difficult time accepting. I have learned that a new situation will arise and if I make a mistake, it's a new mistake. Since I am human, and I'm not perfect, this mistake is only natural. And I have to get myself to ask, "What can I learn from this?" and "How can I not make the same mistake again?"

I am still learning how to not be incredibly difficult on myself when I do make a mistake. I am a person that holds such high standards for myself and has trained myself to have such low standards for everyone else. So, I'm still working through this problem myself. When I finally do realize that I need to stop criticizing myself, give compassion to myself, and focus on a solution to not making the same mistake again; that's when I form many ideas or plans to improving. Some work and some don't, it's a learning process. I keep trying until I find something that works.

The mistakes don't have to be major mistakes, they can be simple or minute. It doesn't matter as long as it's considered a mistake. Trying to defend the mistake by trying to convince yourself that it's not a mistake because…, is not going to be helpful. Justifying the mistake does not make it ok, it's giving in to denial. Know that the first step is acceptance, after that you go on a cycle or process of learning to fix the mistake(s). You end up making yourself a better person, one even other people will value and take you more seriously. You show people that you can be given credibility and can be trusted. That's why It's important to ignore the desire to go into denial. That first step can be the one thing to make a major difference in your life.

An example of a recent mistake I've made is making a comment to a family member that I didn't realize how hurtful it was going to be. At the time I didn't care about anyone else's feelings and was only focused on my own rage. I made a comment that was lashing out irrationally and it hurt this person's feelings more than I could have imagined. I realized later how hurtful I was to this person and acknowledged that I was wrong to react based on my emotion and I did not mean to cause so much distress. I could say that because it is true. I was being real, and honest.

There is a lot of tension and drama in my family and it frustrates me so much but even so, they are my family and the last thing I want to do is to hurt them. As a young child, I learned early on that family is really all I have and all I need. If I have my family, I can be happy. So, the tension and drama are an obstacle that I have to work around because my family matters to me. The family member that I irrationally lashed out at listened to me and could tell that I was being real and being genuine, there was a new understanding from both of us afterwards that has helped us to learn from the situation so we can work together to help each other out. As a result, it's learning from the mistake.

Which is another point I want to make. You don't have to learn from your mistakes alone. If there is someone that can assist you, let them. Two heads are better than one, this other person may have another viewpoint that sheds light on a new idea that could work out. Let people reach out to you to assist you in learning from mistakes. And if the time ever comes that someone could use a hand you can reach out to them, to assist them as well. It's a way of seeing people as human, and yourself as human; and accepting everyone for themselves and not criticizing the differences. Just because it's different doesn't make it wrong, it just makes it a different viewpoint that could be a cool new way for you to see things.

Because Trauma…

Chapter Three

train of thought derailing, now

you can't see past the pain, now

Response: "It's not socially acceptable…"

Living in society there are standards. Sometimes things going on internally in the mind can clash with what is socially acceptable. In other words, it is out of the social norm. Sometimes there is a frustration and panic to survive in society and mimicking social cues and behaviors to blend in, become a tool to keep going and not draw attention. But when there are thoughts, emotions, or experiences that do not line up with societies standards the natural reaction is to not make it known to other people. It becomes a secret that someone has become too fearful to acknowledge. That becomes a problem when that information begins to feel like its eating away at you internally. It finds a way to become a problem and put itself on repeat sometimes on a daily basis leading to more anxiety and the person feeling more like a social outcast.

A situation I am dealing with and still working to overcome is more of a possibility and less confirmed through tangible proof. There is no tangible proof but there are years of my own thoughts and feelings towards the issue and the reoccurring nightmare I have had for over twenty years. It dates back to when I was around six years old with my half-sister. She was 17 at the time and she had lived with my mom and dad for about a year before moving out. My half-sister is my dad's daughter and her mother, from my understanding, was not the best mother. My parents would pick her up when she was just two years old to have their time raising her and she would always be a mess. When my parents got her, they brought her home and the first thing they did was get her cleaned up. Then they had to trim her nails because it looked like they haven't been since the last time my parents had her and did it themselves. They had to make sure she was healthy and doing ok. Her mother had some issues that I am not fully aware of but know it was along the lines of substance or alcohol abuse. She was very rude to my dad and my mom and always was trying to tell my half-sister that she is her family and my mom, step-brother and I were not. Around when I was six my parents noticed a real change in me. I was a very happy kid but shortly after my step-sister moved in it all changed. I became a nightmare to my parents. I have a cousin that is just under a year older than me and when we were that young, she would love to be a good cousin and give hugs to be friendly. Before my half-sister moved in, I was ok with it, but after a few months; I squirmed away and showed that I didn't like it. It's when I developed a serious personal space issue. Even now, over 20 years later, I'm not someone that will be open to hugs or getting very affectionate.

I don't have any memory of what really happened when I was six. I do know that I am very uncomfortable around my half-sister, I can't tolerate rap music because it's all she listens to and I have a specific memory of going up the stairs in the home and hearing my half-sister blasting her rap music that had language that a child wouldn't understand or like; and I remember just wishing she would turn it off because I thought it was terrible music. I also know she's an alcoholic and the type of person that has a full-time job but spends the nights drinking. She has been married once and it didn't work out, her choices in relationships are not great and she has had much trouble with boyfriends.

I understand I am leading readers into this and a direct explanation of what I think happened, is needed. That's why I understand any frustrations when I say I am not going to say. If I could actually say I would, unfortunately it's still something that I am trying to work through and be able to admit to myself. It's just too difficult for me right now. I need more time to work through things, process things, and move to acceptance. I need more time, going at my own pace, and in the future,

I hope to be able to speak about this. I can say that one of the reasons I have trouble saying anything is I understand how socially unacceptable the information is. My generation has learned that you just don't talk about this. The generation after me has really gotten into the "Me Too" movement and I am all for that but first I need time to be ok with it myself.

Sally Taylor

Chapter Four

a glimmer of hope, so fleeting.

Heart heavy, eyes steady,

Response: "It's too emotionally painful…"

Some things are difficult to process or accept. Some things are very emotionally painful. When another person says or does something that hurts on an emotional level, sometimes shaking your core values; it can be very difficult to deal with. Everyone has their own limits on a number of things, whether it be values, beliefs, ideas, rules; whatever it is, there is a boundary or line that each person has set that will not cross. It has to do with a person's ethical standpoint.

Some people are fine with pushing their limit to an extreme but others not so much. It doesn't make one person wrong and the other right, it just means one person is more comfortable with going so far in something than another, and that is what is so great about this world and the people living on it, if everyone had the same limits then life for people would be so dull. Having differences in everyone makes everyone unique and has value in their own way and each person's perspective has a different view point that can be a creative new way to see the world.

With so much diversity in the world, it makes the world not so divided with two sides but instead has so many sides. In many cases, there is no one right answer, there can be many. Which is great for people to find the options they have and decide for themselves what they think would work out best for them. We have choices. And I know I've gone on a tangent here but I do have a point.

With so many options and people having their own limits, learning to respect that this person's limit is not as extreme as yours, and it's ok because their limit for something else may reach more extreme for one's selves' comfort. Some people have a more difficult time dealing with something that another person did or said that hurt on an emotional level. It takes an unknown amount of time for the person hurt to recover from that, sometimes taking the person who hurt, needing their own time to recover as well.

My own situation has to do with a close family member of mine, my mother. For most of my life, if not my whole life; I have tried to communicate to her to tell her something is wrong. It can be situations so simple and unimportant or something very important, it doesn't matter; I am not heard. As a child I tried to communicate to my mother that my father was beating my step-brother and me. One time my mother was changing my step-brother's diapers and saw the bruises. She questioned my father and he just dismissed it. If she had heard me when I told her dad was beating us, she could easily connect the dots.

Years later my mother, step-brother, cousin and I were spending time together. I don't remember the specifics of what started the conversation, but the topic of my step-brother and I being beaten by our father came up; and my cousin said something that really struck me. She said that when my step-brother and I would go over to her house to spend time there she would ask how we were when we got there and my step-brother and I usually responded that we were beaten by our father again, as if it was just the normal thing. My cousin was conflicted and concerned, but didn't know what to do or say. My mom who heard the whole conversation responded by saying she had no idea that is what our dad was doing and if she knew she would never have let it happen.

I could have responded to that by saying that my step-brother and I communicated to her for so many years as it was happening, and if you would have actually heard your kids tell you their father is beating us, actually paid a little attention, you would have known then and we would not have endured years of being beaten. I could have said that, I wanted to, I was just too angry with the response she gave and couldn't even process it then.

Unfortunately, that is not the only situation where I was not heard by my mother. In seventh grade an old friend tried to kill me by choking me and I went to my mom distraught and I was ignored left to figure it out alone. Years later I was still tormented by the incident in seventh grade and I spoke up about it to my mother who responded that she had no idea it ever happened. She also responded another time before that saying she didn't know what to do since we were on a long-distance school field trip, that took a lot for the both of us to go on. She didn't want to rock the boat with the other parents by looking into it.

My concern in these situations is she remembers me going to her in full tears, broken up by my best friend just trying to kill me; and she's playing this game of whether or not to be truthful or play ignorant. How could any parent not look into the situation if their kid just went through such a moment where a friend tried to kill them? If the kid is lying then look into it to teach a lesson in not lying, if not; the situation is not ok and something needs to be done or be changed.

It doesn't matter what I say, I have accepted that she is not going to hear me. Doesn't matter if it is physical abuse or attempted murder, she doesn't actually care to give me the time to hear me and take me seriously. It's one of the more emotionally painful things I am currently dealing with. Accepting that my mother says she cares but her actions speak so much louder, and they tell me she doesn't.

Currently my mother and I are in a very tense relationship. I've heard from a number of people that the route I am taking in life, being so emotionally invested in family and trying to make peace; is going to result in my death. It was destroying me. For over a year I lost my appetite and barely ate, something I'm still struggling with. I knew I had to take some major steps away from the drama between my mom and I. It went against one of my core values but I understood that the core value I developed early on in life was wrong.

On January 17, 2020; I had my last chat with my mother and January 18 was the first day that I didn't reach out and accepted that I needed space to figure things out. As I am writing this, it's February 17, 2020. The extreme emotional pain I had and the anger I had building because of my mother has dissolved and turned into disappointment. There are still very difficult days where I feel compelled to reach out to my mother but I have learned to get busy when I notice I'm struggling. It also helps to know that my mother hasn't reached out herself because she's using a silent treatment tactic to try to wait me out until I give up and "crawl back" to her. It's unfortunate that it's going to backfire on her because it's what I need for me to really see that a relationship with her is not a smart idea now. I'm hoping that in the future I can have a mother daughter relationship with her again, but it won't be a moment before she figures out the guilt she's been fighting with and truly wants to make things right and not for the sake of her own agenda purposes.

    One of the last few real conversations I had with my mother that left me in tears a few months ago; I thought would be a turning point in our relationship, for the better. I was mistaken, but am surprised that she actually heard me for once in her life. I was in tears when talking with her, so fed up and frustrated with how things have spiraled so far into wrong. She was asking what was so wrong that led to that moment and I expressed to her how I am not heard, even when it matters most.

I used my dad beating my step-brother and me, as well as my friend years ago that tried to choke me. I told her that those actions were so wrong and when I tried to go to my mother to help fix the corrupt actions, because I was just a child and had no power to fix myself; I was ignored, dismissed, and left to deal with it alone.

I tried to express how young children look to their parents as their protectors when growing up but for me, my dad beat me and my mom let it happen by turning her back and ignoring it. I didn't feel protected or safe. She got the message; because sometime after I left, she communicated with dad and finally asked him if what I said was true. And for the first time, dad owned up to it.

When she told me about the conversation, she had with dad a little over a week after, I was shocked. It took me days to be able to begin to process it. My hopes of things getting better was dashed because nothing changed for the better. It got worse. And I bowed out of her life to finally focus on mine.

Sally Taylor

Chapter Five

and wide.

You pray for that moment

Response: "I don't trust my own judgement or feelings sometimes."

I lack confidence and self-esteem. I'm aware of how much of a problem it is. I've gone years not trusting my own intuition because when I was growing up, I learned from my parents that; it's either wrong or not possible to be able to do what anyone can do with a highly developed intuition. My parents don't understand someone capable of high intuition and they don't accept it. The expectation to do or act along the same ways as them, has been the key struggle and difference between my parents and me.

I had to adapt early on with my parent's standards of the norm because if I didn't; I'd get a response of, "I'm hallucinating," "I'm just being crazy," "That's stupid," or any array of responses along those lines. I learned not to trust my intuition or my own judgement early on and it eventually became the natural thing to do because I lost so much confidence and self-esteem. It destroyed me. After moving out on my own, I started working on trusting my intuition and judgement more. I began relying on it more and so far, it's been the best idea. I still have a long way to go with building up more confidence and self-esteem but it's something I'm working on daily.

There were times where they thought it was cute or neat, how I could speak up on some strange but true fact as if out of nowhere. They'd ask how I knew it or where I learned that and I could usually recall when or where I learned the fact and explain more on it. It's cute at age six or nine, but when you're older the fun of it fades and I'm now just a slightly annoying weird fact collector.

I will get there with building my confidence and self-esteem, and as far as trusting my feelings; that's a whole other situation. I can easily understand another person's emotions and feelings towards any issue. I can emphasize so well that it's an automatic, natural function. But that's other people. When it comes to understanding my own feelings and emotions, same rules do not apply. It's like my own feelings and emotions are like deciphering a foreign language. I don't understand my own feelings and emotions and many times don't realize what I am feeling until someone asks why I have a look of whatever emotion.

This lack of understanding of my own emotions and feelings may also play a role in how I forget to take care of some of the most basic needs. I tend to forget to eat.

Either I'm working on something and don't realize I'm getting hungry or I don't understand that I haven't eaten in over 30 hours and even though I'm mentally struggling and have no appetite, I need to eat something. I've been so stuck in my own thoughts that, one time I forgot to eat for over two days.

My personality is so geared on making sure everyone else is ok before checking with myself. It's because if someone around me is not ok, I'll know it, I'll experience it too. With the lack of confidence and self-esteem, I'm not great at stepping forward to help others. I'm quite fearful. It doesn't help when I am fearful of experiencing another person's strong upsetting or negative emotions. I haven't found a way to not get swept up in their emotions. I'm currently researching to find ways to protect or guard myself so I can help without being consumed with their emotions.

An unusual but great example I have for picking up so quickly on another's emotions is the many times I attempt to grocery shop. I'd just enter the parking lot looking for a parking spot and would instantly be uncomfortable and have a shift in mood. Many times, I'd be too freaked out and uncomfortable to stay and would either drive to another grocery store or just go home and save the shopping for another day. I finally forced myself to park and take a moment to try to understand what was going on, and that's when I'd see the shopper with a cartful leaving the building, pushing the cart with one hand as they held their phone to their ear and ranted and raged. I couldn't even see into the building to know that someone was having a bad ranting day, yet I picked up on it before I even knew what was really going on.

It freaks me out often and I'm working on trying to understand and work with this strange situation, I seem to naturally collect emotions; even when they are not my own. An extreme opposite situation is when I'm interning at a local church for video production and the people in the room are happy, grateful, loving, worshiping, and joyful; I've picked up on the room quickly and would tear up from the amount of happiness or joy or would get overwhelmed with all good emotions. Sounds great but sometimes it's too much, I lose focus and am not effectively doing what I'm there to do. I get caught up with everyone else in what the mood is in the room and I'll lose track of where I'm at in the lyrics when running the slides and could end up one or two slides behind.

What does all this mean for a traumatic situation? Growing up in a family that expects you to behave or function in a way that's not natural for yourself is difficult, and when pressured or criticized to change to their methods and functioning over many years; it becomes more of a bad situation where your own family can't accept you for you and expect you to change the very normal and natural way you function, rather than try to understand or accept. It's difficult and leads to many years of criticism and comments from parents drilling you on how to do something better when there's no one right answer and you need to be able to function in your own ways. Speaking along the lines of intuitive, details don't always need to take top priority and expecting someone so naturally talented with being conceptual and abstract to focus on every minor detail is brutal. What if it was the other way around, and the expectation was to be as conceptual and abstract and there were such major criticisms on being too detail focused? If the tables were turned, would that be, ok? No, not really; there's a give and take on both sides where both differences would be best to find a middle ground.

It doesn't just have to be with intuition, it could be a situation where someone easily expresses emotion too well and is expected to be very reserved and composed with their emotions, the point is the struggle when there's lack of acceptance for you just being you. In any situation or reason why there's criticism; it's not ok and very difficult to deal with and can lead to a traumatic situation.

Sally Taylor

Chapter Six

of peace.

Pause. Wait. Not here, not now.

Response: "I'm afraid I'll have my last meltdown…"

Disclaimer, this chapter gets into the topic of suicide. If you are dealing with these thoughts yourself, skipping this chapter would likely be best. This chapter is not promoting suicide but rather exploring the thought process of someone who's dealt with it. If you are dealing with these thought patterns, find someone to reach out to for support or help. Skip this chapter.

There is a constant fear that I'll get to upset or something would happen and it's more than I can manage. Where I'd give up on life and help myself to my end. I've been in some very low moments and situations where I could have tried convincing myself to just give up and it would have been so easy to take that final step. Either I'm too driven to beat the odds, I'm too stubborn to take the easy way out, or it's actually an act of God that prevents me from making that final decision; I'm not sure but what I do know is I'm here now writing this book after so many moments where it would have seemed better to make the final decision.

I know when I get too stressed or worked up and in a full emotional spiral, I'll do what I can to find a way to get somewhere where I can be alone. It's not to make the final decision but to just get away from other people to process and take time for myself, I'm very much an introverted person and when I'm so worked up, I don't want to be around other's but rather want to hang out alone in my own space. Take my time to recover and process through whatever I was dealing with. I also know when I'm that worked up, I fall into this pattern of shutting down, I stop communicating and isolate myself not just externally by getting away from people but I slip into my own head so much that time goes by that may seem like minutes but really, it's hours. I get lost in my own head, my own thoughts; and that's where I feel safe and thrive.

I know the topic of suicide raises a lot of red flags for medical professionals or just anyone that hears about it. I get that, I'm not trying to raise red flags here just trying to explore the thought process of someone dealing with this. Honestly, I don't have the best personal experience, I have the occasional thought when I'm in serious dark moments but never go so far as to give those thoughts any value, power or say. I know at the time I'm struggling though something difficult and it's not forever, and I just need to bide my time or grit though it and things will work out.

I do, however, have a friend that struggled more with suicidal thoughts. And it was difficult in my position to talk her down. I wasn't in the best place myself to have anything to say about suicidal thoughts and I was just a kid in high school having no training or understanding in talking someone out of suicide.

I attended a private high school where the entire class base of the school was maxed at 140 students. It was a small school with classrooms ranging from 3 to 10 students. I remember many times I'd be pulled out of class by another teacher who asked if I could go sit with my friend and talk to her because she was skipping class and refusing too corporate. I'd usually find my friend in the courtyard, she'd usually be doing something along the lines of self-harm, like cutting. I'd have to sit with her and try to get through to her by trying to get her to communicate to me what was going on. She'd talk a lot of family problems and would quickly move to thinking about making the final decision in suicide.

I learned quickly with the conversation patterns how much I could get through to her or not, sometimes there would be nothing I could say that could help and I'd have real concerns of losing my friend. Many times, I could chat with her and hear what she needed to say and would work on discussing what she could do instead of making the final decision and what she needed to get back to class. My recant of these situations seem simple but it took time and treading carefully on what questions I asked and what I said, to not upset her more or lead her into the wrong direction.

Again, I'm just a high school student also dealing with difficult mental health issues, I wasn't qualified or trained to deal with this stuff but when it came to my friend and a teacher specifically pulls me from class, I'm doing what I can to help. But it takes a toll on me. Especially the times where I was too late to communicate and hear my friend.

One time in particular, scared me the most. It was early morning and classes hadn't started yet. I found my friend near the parking lot, sitting on the stairs leading to the building. She was already self-harming by digging deeper into her wrist where she previously was cutting. I was concerned because she was getting very deep and I didn't know if she'd knick something she wouldn't survive from. I started by trying to get her to open up to me and tell me what was going on but quickly found out she was in a mindset that I couldn't get through to. She had already spiraled so deep that I wouldn't be able to reach her.

I was afraid, I knew I needed to find a teacher or someone to get my friend help but I was too afraid to leave her side because I thought that if I left her that moment she'd make that final decision, especially if she knew I was leaving to get her help. There were no teachers around to get their attention, and trust me; I frantically looked for someone. All I knew to do was to stay there with my friend trying to get through to her while knowing I had no chance this time, and praying that she wouldn't end her life right there. The first bell to get to classes began and she surprised me by heading to class, I followed behind to make sure she made it before finding a teacher or someone who could get her the help she needed.

At the time, I was so concerned and focused on being there for my friend who could potentially end her life; I didn't care about any possible legalities if she actually went through with it. It wasn't even a passing thought, my friend was really struggling and needed someone; I wasn't going to leave her because of any legalities or concerns for me being there as she made that final decision. I was trying to guide her from that even when I knew I wasn't equipped, trained or skilled enough to talk someone out of that much darkness.

It's been more than 15 years since those moments in high school with my friend really struggling. She's since moved away with her family and I haven't heard anything from her in more than 10 years. I still go through days where I'm brought back to those moments where I had to talk my friend out of suicide. Mainly when I'm with others who are talking about troubling family or friend situations, it brings me back to the challenges with my friend. I still have nightmares over losing friends to suicide and it usually plays out with me trying to help but failing.

The moment where I knew I had no chance at getting through to my friend and I feared for her life was so traumatic and difficult for me that I still am plagued by flashbacks and nightmares. But I was there for my friend and she survived that moment. I did find someone who got her the help she needed. Even after all that, it still haunts me.

Maybe having the situations where I wasn't in the best place mentally, in high school, trying to talk my friend out of suicide; has somehow been helpful for me to know not to go that far myself. There were times where I was struggling and had to lead my friend in advice that I didn't believe, but knew it was because I was struggling and it was still the right thing to say. I didn't believe it, I thought what I was saying was bull-crap; yet it still was helpful to my friend and I still was able to help her be ok and get back to class.

Maybe talking someone out of suicide when you don't believe your own words because you're in a similar boat, is just what is needed to get through to yourself to not make the same choices that another person is trying to make. Maybe helping them and seeing how they are able to continue holds some power in preventing you from making those choices. I'm not entirely sure, I just know I've had serious dark moments where that choice would have been simple and I'm still here today; having not made that choice.

Sally Taylor

Chapter Seven

Panic.

Another round of hurt,

Response: "I don't have the proof or evidence to back this up, I can't accept false information…"

There is no proof to certain situations of my past, no tangible proof at least. All I really have is moments of time missing from checking out that still continue to this day, other people's concern and questions when I don't seem like myself; a reoccurring nightmare that's persistent, and my own untrusting fear of others along with the need for distance.

After years of trying to understand and figure out what I was dealing with, I've established that the situation with time gaps may all be linked to me from age 6. My father had finally leaked information that I was a happy kid until around 6 years old, the same time my half-sister moved in with us and mysteriously moved out one year later.

I still can't get a straight answer from my parents on the reason. There are times when I hadn't questioned my parents on my half-sister but they feel some need to go into a long-drawn-out story to why he moved out and every time the story changes too much to be nothing.

Over the years I've heard so many versions from my parents on why, some ending with her mother being the reason, or she wanted to move in with friends, or it just wasn't working out; but none of which said together in the same story. I've heard so many versions by now that I have no way of determining which is true, if any. I also can't ignore my tension or strain when I have to be around her or even have to hear someone mention something about her. I can't ignore the fact that she's dealing, in her own way with something through drinking, I see her as an alcoholic now. When I do see her, what little I'm around her, she's usually got a beer in hand. I don't have a memory of her now without drinking alcohol. I'd go on more about how bad the drinking has spiraled into all wrong by the empty beer bottles and cans scattered around her home, because I've actually seen it, but what would it solve? Instead, all I'll say is she's an alcoholic because she drinks all the time and it's a top conversation on her list of conversations. And it's not because she's a bad person but truly dealing with something.

I still get very unhinged, very upset and struggle to cope. But I've learned how to not check out and get through the moment. I've started using new strategies for coping, many of the old were destructive and unhelpful, so I started new. Some nights I'll go out on late night rant-drives, where it's around midnight and I'm going on a random hour or so drive listening to music, crying, ranting to my steering wheel. Other nights I go on walks, I'll leave my apartment middle of night and just walk in the dark. I have my headphones on and sometimes carry a flashlight, but I'm walking alone to process and burn some pent-up emotional energy. I keep track of my own emotions more, though I'm not great at focusing on myself and my own emotions; they seem so much like a foreign language, I'm still giving more of myself to being mindful of how I actually am. It has helped in combatting those moments of "checking out." It doesn't make life any easier to deal with and I still have days that go completely sideways.

    Some days I'll not realize how upset or troubled I am over something, and it takes a bit of time for things to continually go wrong before I stop and have to ask myself what I'm fighting against with myself, what is bothering me so much that I'm failing at the simplest tasks? Usually that's how it goes, I'm frustrated or upset and trying to accomplish anything goes wrong and continues until I stop myself and force myself to figure out what's bothering me. The point isn't to beat myself up about it but to understand and figure out what I can do to work through it or get past it to continue my day. Sometimes, there's no solution and I have to accept that I need time to just chill and relax then get back to working on what I need to for the day. Projects are prioritized and sometimes projects move to the next day because I needed to take time for myself. It's ok, the project still gets done and I get back on track with things. It's not always necessary to always be productive and make progress on stuff, sometimes stopping to just relax and enjoy chill time can create better productive days going forward.

Some things need tangible proof in order for something to be done, it's generally how the system works for the courts in the United States, I'm sure other countries have something similar along the lines of needing some sort of proof. If you don't have that proof or evidence, then it's hearsay.

Sometimes there's a family secret, one that doesn't have any documentation to act as evidence or proof; and that secret may get buried, hidden from people that may be traumatized by it but don't actually know what it is. In some cases, it may be better not knowing; other's it may be necessary to know. Each family has their own skeletons in their closets, not wanting the rest of the world to know, and not wanting some family to know. The idea behind hiding these secrets was not to create more trouble, but out of fear and many times an attempt to protect.

One way I function is by intuition. It's the most disrespectful function when it comes to tangible proof or details. It's like piecing together a puzzle without all the pieces, thinking they are not necessary and the concept of the puzzle is what matters. Once you know, the details become irrelevant. I'm so natural with my own intuition that I try to argue on details when I don't care about the details. I'd rather reach the results and only give the gist or the concept.

One example was when I was living at my childhood home and I was home alone when at truck pulled up to the front of the house and parked. I was watching TV in the living room and I started hearing a noise as if someone was trying to break into the house by breaking in the front door, which was connected to the living room. I rushed to the door and pulled the curtain covering the window just enough to see a guy trying to break in. He must've seen me because he ran back to his truck and took off down the road.

I called the police who came and started asking about the details. I was more focused on the conceptual story that I couldn't definitively give the color of the truck, it was either white, silver or grey. I don't know I don't care about the color of the truck; the man drove down the road with no exit; just drive that way and you'll find him. The cop didn't appreciate how I struggled to give basic details. But in my own panic and my own uninterest in the details, I didn't stop to focus on every detail I could of the man and his truck.

In this case, because I couldn't give an actual definitive color to the truck, there was lack of evidence and the cop left while the guy in his truck, may have left to try to break into more homes. I hope someone better with details was able to be more helpful to the police and this guy didn't unravel too many lives of homeowners and families.

Because Trauma…

Chapter Eight

another round of screaming

in your own head.

Response: "It's my problem and my responsibility and I don't expect anyone to understand or be burdened by it…"

I know I've had to learn to deal with situations at a very young age that most children don't deal with. I know now I was aware of very few options on dealing with it all. One of them was to give up and pass away, another was to find whatever way I could to make it through. I did speak up when I saw my grandfather turn into what I call a monster, he'd get so angry and I could tell in his eyes he was gone. He'd chase me and my step-brother around the house when he was so enraged, catching us and hitting us with his belt.

Every kid would be horrified by this and I did speak up to my mother, going to her for protection because every kid is supposed to grow up knowing their parents will protect them. I found out that I was unheard, by my mother. It didn't matter how much I tried to communicate the wrong or when she saw the marks on my step-brother, she went to my grandfather and questioned him before hearing her own kid tell her what was going on. My grandfather excused it away as nothing and my mom was none the wiser. I eventually gave up trying to get through to my mother about the abuse because I lost hope that she'd hear me.

One shocking conversation with my mom, step-brother, aunt and I really caught me off guard when I was in my mid-twenties. Somehow the topic of my step-brother and I being hit by our grandfather came up and my aunt mentioned something that concerned her but she didn't know what to do. She said she remembers when my step-brother and I would go to her place to spend the night and my step-brother and I would casually dismiss the abuse by saying we were ok and that our grandfather just was mad and hitting us again; like it was no big deal and it was just the normal.

Even then, my mother paid no attention; she actually laughed it off and dismissed it. It took me being fed up with not being heard for her to finally question my grandfather and ask him if there's any truth behind what I was saying, and for the first time; he owned up to it, I was 29 by then. What I'm getting at with this dragged-out explanation is, I had to learn how to manage on my own at such a young age. I may have found very unconventional methods of coping but I'm still here breathing. I've struggled through more than any child or human should and I've done the majority of it on my own.

I've accepted that my life is my responsibility and I'll find my own way to manage because it's what I've had to do at such a young age. After over 30 years, why should that be any different? I've made it 30 years, now more than ever; my life, my responsibility. I've had to grow up learning that people don't care to hear about the wrongs in life and you have to learn how to manage on your own very quickly, or die trying. Even now, I'm 30 and questioning humanity. I struggle to see good in this world. It may be because I've had to finally call it quits with the relationship between my mother and I and I'm just trying to find a reason to move forward in life. I'm now rejecting all my core concepts of family I grew up with as false and have to quickly adapt to new. It's rough, I'm missing the idea of a good mother-daughter relationship which is something I never actually had. In a way, I'm also kicking myself for not figuring this out sooner.

Because Trauma…

Chapter Nine

You hope that instead,

you find someone not red.

Response: "Saying it makes it more real."

Saying something horrific and tragic happened makes it so much more real. I've hidden behind the illusion of no such wrongs happened by not speaking of them. It was easy for me because I was overwhelmed and had found a way to "check out" and I didn't understand what was really going on. I took an abnormal psychology class in college when I was going for my associates and when I signed up for the class, I made a promise to myself that I wasn't going to diagnose myself with everything out of the book and I was going to be realistic and critical of what caught my attention and if there was something that really bugged me, I'd go ask my psychiatrist to explain or help me understand why or why not it's possible.

I was so misguided in this class but I held true to not diagnosing myself with everything out of the book. The elaborateness of the human mind can make for one issue and if there's a small detail difference, it could make for a different issue; issue meaning mental health concern. I stuck with keeping close eye on a few concerns with some disorders I studied out of the book, but where I mess up is when I hear other people comment and say "that something I say or do seems a lot like…"

I may argue their point at first but that's the same time the spark of doubt and concern starts. I question it and don't even realize I'm on alert looking to prove their point. I've been so great with agreeing with someone and trashing my own thoughts at times, and it's bad when the person I accept the information from may hold little to no truth. I didn't really get much closer to understanding from this class, though I do promote taking psychology classes if you're interested and want to learn from them.

It was years later when I dove into personality theory, that I started making the connections to understanding what I've been dealing with. Sure, it's not yet accepted by the medical community as a valid scientific way to understanding someone's personality, it's still strictly theory; and that's fine. But I can't argue with the results after using this understanding to work on personal development. Sure, I've still got a long way to go but I can see the progress I've made thus far.

It took so much to get to the point of being able to grit through the difficulty of self-development. I was in over my head with depression and anxiety and going through a roller coaster of emotions with family drama. I still am but I've reached an understanding on taking it one step at a time to get to something better. It sucks now, but by actively working towards something better; eventually you'll get there.

I still notice the same old patterns I've been working on breaking spark and it's a daily challenge to not fall back into that trap. I still struggle to confront difficult situations because I'm afraid to admit to them and make them real. I still tend to lean towards shutting down and not talking about it, in hopes that if I don't say anything; maybe it would really be real. This isn't just my own observation but a medical professionals' observation when I've commented vaguely on difficult situations.

I'm currently dealing with a decision where I feel like the worst person in the world because I made a decision to cut ties with the majority of my family. I'm struggling to open up about this to anyone, and this medical professional has noticed this and commented on how I need to not shut down and take a chance to open up to someone to deal with it.

It's not easy for me, every time I open up just a little, I panic after and feel like I've made a mistake opening up; I've created trouble for someone else by sharing, I've burdened someone else. So now, it's bracing myself for every moment that it gets more real and to keep pushing myself forward to the truth and a better outcome. And I still have to give myself a day, occasionally, to be freaked out and horrified and find a way to gather myself enough to keep going.

Sally Taylor

Chapter Ten

With hate.

With anger.

Response: "I'm afraid this will backfire on me..."

I've experienced too well the ramifications of speaking your mind on an unsettling matter and that act of speaking up "blows up in my face" or backfires on me. One example in grade school, before I understood my sense of hearing was a little better, due to being born without the ability to smell; I'd hear classmates talking a decent distance away and would get upset or "bent out of shape" when I heard them criticizing me.

I'm going to give a disclaimer here, I did not make it difficult for my peers to find ways to criticize me; they didn't understand and quite frankly, neither did I. I was a very strange kid growing up and if it was so difficult for me to understand myself, how could I expect anyone else to? That still doesn't make the criticisms any less painful. When I would hear one classmate talking with another about some unethical or immoral behavior, and they just finished making critical remarks about me; I saw fit to inform the teacher or someone of their plan to try to help anyone on the receiving end of their plan.

And yeah, I was upset and wanted them to be held accountable. I learned that informing the teacher would backfire on me very quickly. Because the teacher would go question the students and since it was a plan that would not be appropriate or permitted, the students would lie and say that they never discussed this and there's no way anyone could say I heard them. I could hear how their voices changed when they denied the conversation. I didn't know then but when the sense of hearing is stronger than typical, the inflections in someone's voice when trying to lie or give a less than truthful excuse is not hard to notice. It's a very obvious change that I didn't understand could be difficult for anyone that doesn't have heightened hearing because of the loss of another sense.

Their defense was that they were too far away for me to actually be able to hear and when explaining this to the teacher questioning them, a few times with me nearby, I could see the hateful and even vengeful looks from the students when they got the chance. It was obvious I could hear their conversation and the hateful looks after a teacher questioned them with their voices slightly changing when providing an answer didn't align with the truth, the pitch was a little higher and they spoke in a peppier downplay tone, which is how I describe someone trying to convince someone else everything is ok, good or not true by sounding more chipper, upbeat, innocent, or almost full of themselves.

After a few repeated outcomes with classmates trying to cover their own rear-ends by lying about a conversation I overheard, I learned to not say anything anymore on the conversations I heard where students were going to participate in something wrong. That didn't change, even into college. I remember hearing two students in high school planning out a way to steal food from the lunchroom pantry. It's a room where students don't need the school lunch card to get lunch but can bring cash to buy burgers, fries, and other junk style food. That day when I got in line for lunch, those two students got in line about 10 students behind me, one student with a backpack behind the other waiting as the student in-front grabbed a prewrapped food item and handed it back to the other as he stashed it in the backpack, continuing down the line while grabbing more. It didn't take long for the school to notice the numbers didn't add up, in assessing how much food was gone and how much money they had after the students paid for their meal; the school had much less than what they were supposed to. It led to the school making an announcement to all students that if the stealing does not stop, they'd close down the pantry and all students would be stuck with the standard lunch card and assembly style lunch line. I still didn't speak up; I didn't have to that time; another student also watched the two students stealing the food and had spoken up about it.

My reasoning for not speaking up out of fear of backfire is not solely on my unusual ability to hear much better than typical. It is out of fear because I don't want to speak up and it backfire because someone can't take what I say seriously enough and actually believe I'm spitting out BS or fabricating a complete lie as well. It's the believability factor or lack of. I'm not someone who will spit out complete BS or fake information, it takes time for me to speak up and that's mainly because I'm spending time making sure I mean what I say and it's what I believe is true information, usually after spending so much time looking into it and researching.

To then have someone chalk up what I say as fake, unreliable, or BS; is very insulting and hurtful to me and I'd rather not say anything in hopes that the credibility or believability in me and what I say is not damaged or lost even more. I understand now how pathetic it is for me to silence myself out of fear of people thinking I'm BSing with them. It's something I have yet to overcome and learn to speak up again. It is something I'm currently trying to work on.

The student that did speak up and notify the school about the two students that were stealing actually did the right thing in that instance, the school kept this student anonymous for protective reasons, snitches still are frowned upon these days and can lead to physical harm;

in this instance, the school was prepared to shut down the lunchroom pantry and many students who didn't have a lunch card would either have to get one or bring their own lunch. I was one of those students who didn't have a lunch card. I brought my lunch most days and only went through the pantry on occasion, but losing the pantry would be far more upsetting and difficult for other students who couldn't bring their lunch and for some reason couldn't or wouldn't get a lunch card.

Those are two examples from my own personal experience at school but the concept or idea of speaking up and having it backfire on yourself can be applied to any scenario. You don't have to apply this to just school situations, it can relate to family, work, friends, acquaintances, or even strangers. In regards to traumatic events, one of the worst feeling an individual can have is; if they do find the courage to speak up about the traumatic event and are accused of making it up, lying or fabricating the whole story. That is the same concept of having what you speak up and communicate, backfire on yourself. Only with traumatic events, the hurt is so much worse.

Another very real example is having a relationship or acquaintance with a very manipulative person who would listen to what you have to say only to use as ammunition against you later. Whether it be twisting what you said up so much that it's a false story making you look incredibly horrible, or any other version of using your words against yourself. I've had the unfortunate situation happen with my own mother. I was trying to be very upfront and real about concerns and insecurities I had and she took that as an opportunity to twist everything I said up to feed her new version to my 6-month pregnant sister who is then calling me late one night in an emotional rampage over what our mother told her. It saddens me to this day that my relationship with my sister has not recovered. It was clear that night she didn't care what I had to say, she was glued to the fake story our mother fed her and nothing could change that. The phone conversation ended with me having to accept that my sister is just going to have to hate me for a while until she would be willing to accept her information was not correct. To this day, I'm still waiting.

She's since had her daughter and I've noticed this rift between us grow and push us much more distant. I'm not proud to admit that I no longer feel comfortable or welcome around my sister. I've visited a couple of times since her daughter was born but I had other family there to not have this dead silence. I know in the past I wasn't very open with my sister, to me, it seemed like we were from different worlds. She was very outgoing and loved to party and I enjoyed staying home and reading books or playing games. It was no match for us compared to how distant we are now. I barley utter two words to her when visiting. I don't know how because I can't see or get past my own hurt. I wonder often if she's feeling the same or if she's managing better.

Because Trauma…

Chapter Eleven

With rage.

They don't see you as you, now.

Response: "I've never talked about this before and I don't know how to or where to begin…"

I'm not great with talking about how I feel or my emotions. Mainly because I'd rather focus on other people and what they are dealing with, many times it's to avoid my own emotions. I don't know how to put what I'm dealing with into words and with my fear of trusting someone enough to let them know about what's going on as a leading concern, I don't talk about the deep emotional trouble. Many times, it's because of fear of judgement, fear of not being understood, critical remarks to "get over it" or "it's stupid/crazy to think/feel that."

I've been so focused on what everyone else is dealing with, making sure I find the time for others that I formed a habit in not paying attention to taking care of myself. It tends to go to an extreme where my emotions feel like a tidal wave because I've ignored them so long. It's always been easier for me to ignore them because I don't want to relive whatever is tied to them. I know now that I've kept trying to run to a better future by ignoring my emotions, rather than stop, and wait; to process and deal. It doesn't work. Those tidal wave emotions always push me back farther than I'd like and it's much more difficult to get back on track. I'm not saying I've learned how to deal with whatever emotion I have, I haven't; I just have a starting point of knowing what's not working out.

    Aside from not knowing how to talk about my emotions, I have a difficult time finding the right words to communicate anything. I tend to focus so much on what's acceptable for other people, trying to determine if something would be received well if I were to communicate it and trying to adapt to their language style, within reason; to be able to have a relatability with other's. It sounds exhausting and sometimes it is, but other times its more natural. I think of it as finding other's boundaries to work with and respect in communication. I'm not great at having my own boundaries and would rather know other's and work with that. Typically, the start of a conversation doesn't involve everyone stating their boundaries right off the bat, the topics or content for the reason to communicate is addressed and boundaries are not typically focused on unless there is a problem. I've found a process of understanding someone's boundary just by listening to the conversation and making a mental note of what words they use, what they avoid, what topics in the content are avoided and the overall comfort level for everyone in the conversation. The style of who they are.

If someone is starting out with curse words or rants with more extreme language, their boundary is not drawn before cursing. Though I typically don't join in with their cursing, I still respect that they will curse. If someone is more proper then knowing to stay as close to proper is best. Other factors of how well you know a person can change that, if you're good friends then communicating in your own style tends to be more respected than mimicking your friend.

I have a point to this, finding the boundaries to communicate is key and focusing on something that would be more accepted. If you are always focusing on difficult emotions and generally people like to discuss or focus on more upbeat and interesting topics. Which is also another aspect to boundaries. If someone is not comfortable about talking about certain content, I'm not going to disrespect them by dragging it all up. I'd rather talk about fun upbeat things over darker upsetting things as well.

With focusing on other's so much and putting myself second or even third…or last. I never found a reason to try to understand my emotions or how to deal with them, I didn't care so much for what I was going though because it was too painful and my escape was to focus on how others were doing and completely ignore the painful emotions and everything tied in with them. It works until the tidal wave of emotions hit, then after they subside, I'd continue focusing on everyone else. Unfortunately, it doesn't work out well, and it likely never will. I've since accepted that and am trying to understand myself better to know how to deal with my own confusing emotions better. I'm very behind on this and I know it's going to take some time, but it's necessary.

Sally Taylor

Chapter Twelve

Their anger everlasting.

Long after the event's passing.

Response: "I don't want anyone to see me any differently…"

It's a universal understanding that everyone has their own view of themselves and other people typically have another view. When it comes to traumatic experiences, I stayed silent for a reason. I feared that if I spoke up, the person I spoke up to would view me differently or have an undesired judgement of me. It's only human to want to be seen as strong, weather that be physically, mentally, or emotionally. To have the idea that the situation may be questioned or my emotions or wellbeing, jeopardized just by speaking up about a difficult and traumatic moment is enough for many people to hide that information and see no reason to ever speak of it.

In the time of starting this book and what I've written so far, I started with a list of reasons, or things people say to themselves to not speak up, before adding the context.

When starting with the list I greatly feared people forming an undesired view, opinion, or judgement of me. Now, while writing this chapter, which has been at least year since I created the list; I've learned how impossible it is to avoid someone else having an undesired opinion. People are going to form their own opinions and viewpoints; it happens with everyone, including me. I cannot by any means have any control of what other people form as their opinions. Just like no one can control what opinions I form of them, or anyone for that matter. It's what it means to be an individual. Opinions are diverse concepts that are not always set in stone but sometimes difficult to change. Maybe taking a different approach to understanding why the undesired opinion was formed rather than staying silent and never speaking up about traumatic injustices would have an outcome that is by far better than living in fear of speaking up. I am not condoning causing harm or traumatizing experiences on anyone, but I'm also not condoning staying silent and living in fear of being viewed differently. Maybe having enough individuals speak up on traumatic experiences is enough to spark change, I mean; isn't that how the "Me Too" movement started?

Because Trauma…

Chapter Thirteen

A reoccurring nightmare, for you.

A faded memory, in their journey.

Response: "I've been through enough, bringing it up will only add more emotional pain…"

I don't typically focus on my emotions or what emotional trouble I'm dealing with. Instead, I spend so much time focused on other's emotions because I can understand someone else's much better than my own and I'm distanced a little from others versus my own. I mean, I'm not them but myself. I'd rather deal with someone else's emotions than my own because it's easier. With my emotions seeming more like a foreign language to myself, I struggle to put how I'm feeling into words to communicate.

Many times, I avoid my own feelings to not deal with them. So, communicating what I'm feeling is so difficult and even painful. I don't typically want to communicate what I'm feeling because it's my way to avoid the pain or difficult emotions. I now understand based on my own personality; talking about past experiences that has to do with emotions is a challenge for me to find good to communicate on. Typically, I'm remembering the past that surrounds traumatic events or bad situations that was very troubling.

Another way of putting this is I've been through some tough situations; many have said it was very traumatic. I get it, I have. I know this because I've spent years trying to out-run my own emotions towards my past. But in doing so, I find myself not focusing on my emotions at all and instead focus on others' emotions. I've always been afraid that if I stop to let my own emotions catch up, it will be too much to deal with.

But here's the catch, no one can out-run their emotions for their entire life. Trust me, I've tried and failed in my late 20's. The thing about dealing with past emotions, you can't move forward and be a better person until you do. Surprisingly enough, I've ran towards the future while trying to out-run my emotions hoping to just continue to be steps ahead so I'd never have to deal with them, but I've got a whole army behind me now that may not be as fast as me, but eventually tiering out is a given and that army of emotion is going to eventually close that gap. Then it's a flood of bad emotions hitting and when there's enough of it, there's no chance of keeping that under wraps. Sometimes, the impossible struggle begins.

Unfortunately, my family got to see that in my late 20's into my early 30's. I realized that I'd never escape the emotions I had been avoiding for so long and would never be able to get to a better mindset, life, or ability to function; until I confronted all the past traumatic events, I was holding onto through all the emotions I had out-run for years. I made the choice to stop running and just let it all catch up, hoping I could withstand the rush of horrible emotions hit me all at once. I don't recommend this, trust me; it was a horrible decision. It led to me lashing out at my family so frustrated, traumatized and angry about everything. I pushed them away while confusing them by asking them to be there for me and support me. I saw myself as an explosion of emotions that didn't care who would be in the blast zone. I wanted to care, but couldn't; not at that time.

    I struggled desperately to keep everything together all while the world around me seemed to fall apart, but it was only me; my choice, my own emotions, my issues that were released in the most explosive form of emotions. In the end, it cost me my mother's side of the family, my step-brother to act like I don't exist, and my mother and father unable to get through to me to help nor knowing how to because it was just too much. Currently, I'm still dealing with the blast of emotions, I'm on the downswing but it's still not even close to a resolution. I haven't spoken with my mother's side of the family since July and now is just three days before Christmas. My step-brother won't communicate with me and I'm at the point of seeing the brilliance in that, I wouldn't want to speak with myself if I were her. My parents are just exhausted by everything, since they both don't understand having a child that "wears their heart on their sleeve" and easily expresses emotions rather than keep their emotions to themselves in a very, what I call controlled and restricted manner. It's not I'm just not great at keeping how I feel to myself like my parents.

    Letting all the past emotions I've tried to out-run definitely has been far too much. The emotional pain is at an all-time extreme. I feel like I've drowned in my emotions for over a year now and that there will be no end to the pain. But that's just what I feel. Logically, I can look back and see the progress. I know now it's not very easy to see and it seems like it's actually much worse but that's how it is when you're in the eye of the storm. Which is where I am with everything. I've made it to the very worst of my past traumatic events and am now working through them. The only way I've been able to keep going is by focusing on the path ahead or my goal/mission and keep checking to see the end of this storm. Basically, see the better future where I've worked through all the difficult past situations and have much more stability in my life.

    It's been agonizing, getting up every morning to go to school or go to an internship for school and feeling like I've died inside because the depression has spiraled into something beyond awful. I've started seeing it as high functioning agony. By using the terms high functioning depression with emotional agony. I wish I could just stay home and hide in my apartment talking to no one and just disappearing from existence, it has taken more time in the morning just to get myself motivated to just get out of bed and start the day. By keeping in mind, the goal of graduation and that I have to get up and start the day to pass the semester to get closer to the goal of graduation, I've managed to drag myself out of bed, get up and ready every morning. This fall semester has also been the busiest semester with an internship of 22 hours a week as well as three classes, one of which, had very demanding projects where I filmed over four weekends and drove a total of 18 hours just to get to the four filming locations. After filming I had to also edit the 20+ hours of audio and video to create a segment that ended up being only 6 minutes 45 seconds, total run time. I couldn't risk taking a day and just stay in bed. The classes were far too important for the end goal of graduation. I found a way to just grit through it and keep focused on graduation so I'd be able to just roll with the day and keep working on projects and the internship. Of course, having an internship that I actually liked and wanted to be there for definitely helped. Working with a great upbeat and fun group of people in video production was definitely one of those moments where you find the rare pearl in the shell.

Because Trauma…

Chapter Fourteen

Their fear leading their way.

They are lost, misguided,

Response: "I'm ashamed of the whole situation and too ashamed to talk about it…"

Have you ever felt embarrassed about something? Maybe someone notices a weakness you have and they focus on it a little too much for your comfort. What about feeling ashamed? I've always seen that as a little more intense than embarrassed, but on a tangent. With ashamed, there's a higher level of guilt added. Weather that guilt is from being at fault or not. Guilt is just an emotion after all, there is not logical basis required.

For traumatic situations feeling ashamed is not an uncommon feeling. There's fear to say anything and feeling bad or guilty for not; or guilt for any number of reasons depending on the situation. Maybe someone knows another person is at risk of the same traumatic event and the guilt is from not speaking up to help themselves and the other person from the same fate. Whatever the reason may be, feeling ashamed is an obstacle that is so challenging for someone to speak up about a traumatic event or work through it.

A situation I've been through myself is feeling ashamed to speak up about an abusive situation I found myself in many years ago. I was in middle school and since my parents nor the school system understood what was going on with me, they had hired someone to follow me around to observe and keep an eye out for anyone that would be bullying. To give some insight, this was just before the whole movement of MeToo and the focus on how bad it is for kids to be bullied in school, I believe I was a few years ahead of that time. The school system didn't have a plan in place for students who were bullied so much and were maybe falling behind or dropping out because of it. So, maybe I was a gunnie pig at an attempt to understand, maybe not. I was taking a restroom break and had made it into a stall with the individual (also female) hanging out waiting for me to finish my business when a small group of 2-4 students walked in the bathroom. Their idea of fun was to try to kick the stall door open, the very one I was in, and trying to use the bathroom. The situation ended up with me bracing my feet against the stall door as the small group brutally attacked the door to get it open while I begged, cried and screamed at them to stop. Eventually they left. I still needed to finish using the restroom so I silently broke down into tears, while still in the stall trying to finish. Then I hear someone in the bathroom who had been standing there the entire time, the group attacked the stall door. It was the individual who was supposed to follow me around and observe anything that may be bullying activity. This person had been there the entire time just letting it all happen, and did nothing. Then decides that it's a good idea to tell me to hurry up because it's time to get to class a couple of moments (at most) after this group left.

One of the requirements of this individual was to document or write anything of significance during the day, the situation with the small group was definitely of significance. Years later my parents had a copy of all the notes taken and, when I was moving out into my own apartment the notes made their way to my apartment with the storage tub of old school stuff. I read through the notes looking specifically for the time when the small group was attacking the stall door and this individual had decided to omit an entire hour before, after, and during that moment; from the notes. I hadn't worked through that event so I was horrified by this individual's bad judgement call on leaving out everything with this situation and still, letting it all take place back then as they just stood by and watched.

I was embarrassed and ashamed to say anything about the situation with the group attacking the stall door, but I thought this individual would make the right call to inform someone or at the very least include it in the notes they were hired to write. I couldn't say anything for years because it was so horrifying for me and I truly was ashamed to speak up. At the time, I was a young kid that had no value in what I said, that's why they had this individual follow me around to observe, to be able to verify what I was saying and dealing with. Yet this very person decided to ignore and even omit the very horrific situation as if it never happened. When my own voice holds no value and the person hired to speak up on my behalf and verify what I was saying decides to omit the situation, I didn't see where I had any chance with saying anything on this very traumatic and even embarrassing moment. I was ashamed so I stayed silent for many years, and didn't see how saying anything would help in any way.

Sometimes an emotion has power over someone. Whether it be fear, anger, or feeling ashamed, even very good emotions like feeling happy, overjoyed or in love. Regardless, emotions don't hold logical basis but people tend to sometimes let their emotions make decisions that are not always the best course of action. It's not saying anything bad upon the person, it happens; especially if there's a traumatic event tied into it. I'm noticing all the poor decisions I've made in past traumatic situations where my emotions called the shots and any logical basis was not factored in. It's something I'm still working on, and will continue to work on for many years to come.

Finding a way to realize your emotions are calling the shots and seeing no logical path in decisions is the best way to start to change the course of actions but wanting to work through traumatic situations and take your own power back is a must, first. Being willing to speak up about any wrong and not being afraid or ashamed to do so is something that's really important to helping yourself and maybe even helping others who could be facing the same fate as you. Could there be any greater gift than to take your voice, your power and use it to help yourself and someone else who may be at risk of the same traumatic situation?

Because Trauma…

Chapter Fifteen

into thinking, their action

was a reaction, justified.

Response: "I haven't processed this myself and I need time to, I don't have a good answer yet..."

I'm best at taking time to process something before I respond or give an answer to someone, especially when it comes to something that I'm invested in, been directly hurt by or something needing a thought-out answer or response. I thrive when I get to take time to go process something then return with this great insight or response. I've caught myself spending so much time doing this and it's something that's so natural that I don't even realize how often I slip into this processing mode and shut down, sticking to only my thoughts.

I've always had trouble understanding how someone could give an answer or response to someone when they haven't put the thought into it. For me, that answer or response does not have the quality to it to be as useful as a thought that took time to process through and give a very real, detailed answer. I almost don't trust answers that are blurted out with no real thought to the details of the answer. I may not directly question the validity of the response but I'm definitely processing questions like if I can trust that answer, how much of the answer is actually useful, how much of the half-effort answer is useless for what I need in the answer, or how valid is the answer?

There are exceptions, when I know I'm asking something that another individual has spent many years on, whether it be a job, specific skill or even processing a life situation; not as much thought would be needed in an answer at the time because the thought was already put into the answer. An example I have is when I was in my video production class. I had an idea for a specific camera shot and asked my professor if there was a way to make that camera shot work and what the best way would be. My professor has spent more than twenty years of personal experience in filmmaking as well as teaching at the campus for almost ten, he gave a very quick and natural response like it took nothing to answer. He had enough experience to just know, the shot wouldn't work out and included asking me more questions to fully understand what I was trying to get and giving real examples to why it wouldn't work.

But to my professor, it almost seemed like an automatic answer that really didn't require much thought, only because he's tried shots like that in the past and has the experience to back up why it doesn't work out and that's a profession, he's spent at least 20 years on. He actually knows this stuff and has lived it for so many years, it's like common sense to my professor. Whereas, asking another student the same question, I'd prefer a thought-out answer and not something that they just give a quick simplified response to. Which with this example it would be my mistake to ask another student, expecting a thought-out high-quality answer, when this student doesn't know as much as my professor on filming; since we're learning the same material and have about the same experience level.

I have always lived by if someone wants me to answer something, could be personal could be general; I try to think out and give the best, real answer I can. It's what I naturally do and I don't need to think about thinking it out. I struggle more to give a response that doesn't have any effort or meaning to it, I almost consciously have to be aware and focused on not giving a good answer; and I typically fret about it afterwards or feel bad about the answer I gave.

When it comes to traumatic experiences, many times there's a moment of shock where I can't say anything and need to process through the situation after the fact to really understand what was going on. I need to understand the deeper questions like why it happened and what could I have done to prevent the event or have a better outcome. They are a list of just a few of the many questions I need to process through and form answers to in order to have a better understanding myself. If I don't get that time to process through, I likely wouldn't answer or give an answer of I don't know or I don't understand because I'd rather give that than give a random answer that may be very different later, after I've processed through. It then seems like I was lying earlier to go against what I initially said and that's not really the case, I just couldn't devote enough time to think out the best or most truthful answer to give to the question.

    I've been in conversations before where I've been asked to answer to something and I've declined by saying I hadn't processed much myself to form a great response. I was asked to answer or respond anyways and out of respect for the other person, have responded but I always feel uncomfortable or unhappy with my response; because I'm unsure of my response. But, if I'm asked, I will give an answer or response; even if I'm unhappy with doing so. I will tend to clarify my hesitation first.

Sally Taylor

Chapter Sixteen

Not cruel, not heartless.

Being hateful, creating

Response: "I shouldn't have to answer or defend the situation or my reaction…"

This relies on mainly emotions or actions in response to a difficult or traumatic situation. Traumatic experiences are just that, traumatic experiences. If you've ever been in a situation that is considered a traumatic experience, no one should ever expect you to defend how you feel.

Thinking back to a very real situation with the 9/11 attacks, I was in middle school and watched as the world seemed to stop and watch as the horrors that unfolded when the planes full of passengers turned to fly into the pentagon, twin towers and make an attempt towards the capital. I got a great realization that day that I'm just one person as I watched my classmates and teachers all watch with very real hurt, panic, and concern in their eyes.

I cannot begin to explain what was going on with myself but all I could think to do was to offer assistance by walking classmates to the office so they could call home to be with family. In those moments, it didn't matter to me who you were; bully or good friend, if you needed an escort and an ear to rant to while making your way to the office. I volunteered.

I don't know how many trips I made to the office that day, and I don't really care either; what mattered was focusing my attention on whomever needed it at the time. No one was ever expected to explain themselves on how they were feeling, when the 9/11 attacks happened; it was a very traumatic experience for so many and watched as people set differences aside to help support one another. Which is speaking only on behalf of everyone that was in my school at the time because I was there, I know; and can't really speak on behalf of anywhere else.

It was enough for me to see how people can set aside any daily concerns among one another to be a helpful support during such a difficult time, that's what mattered to me then. I'm in no way trying to minimize the 9/11 attacks, so many were lost and it's very tragic. The point is, even during such tragic moments people still can work together and help one another; even if you don't get along with your neighbor, you and your neighbor are still in the same boat at that time.

The same goes for any traumatic experience, defending your feelings in these matters should never be an issue. Yet sometimes when someone feels isolated or alone on a traumatic experience, not like the 9/11 attacks but a situation that they've experienced on their own; it's difficult to not feel defensive and want to protect and even defend your emotions surrounding whatever difficult situation.

Sometimes it feels like there's lack of understanding because you've dealt with it alone, and the fear of being judged wrongly or criticized for how you've felt or acted plays a serious role in being defensive. After going through such a difficult situation, there's hurt and concern with being hurt again; especially so soon.

There's no shame in reaching out to find support. Finding a group of friends or community that you can lean on and get support is the best self-care solution. Being around people who can be supportive or just toss around jokes to lighten the mood is far better than venturing into any emotions afterwards alone. Many times, the difficult and even harmful emotions proceed, like depression, anger and hate.

But who am I to say anything on overcoming fear to find the support after a traumatic experience? Currently, I'm just another nobody, typing on a computer, in my apartment, highly concerned about my family relationships and the very concept of the family foundation falling apart. It's the most difficult pain of depression I've ever dealt with, and I am in some ways, dealing alone.

It troubles me, that I don't have my own family to lean on for support; yet I've pushed myself to focus on college courses and an internship class that's required for graduation. And that's where I found my support. I noticed early during the internship that I'd get excited to go be a part of the internship, where I get to work with a video production team at a church that adapted amazingly to the pandemic.

I know the individuals I work with at the internship don't quite understand how much they've been a great support for me, I don't really bring up the family drama; because it's not necessary. Just being there, enjoying the time with great individuals, doing what I love and am in school for; that's really all I need as far as support. Getting a few hours out of the day three times a week to go have fun with video production and set aside any life issues outside the internship is an amazing help in finding the support and peace needed.

I'm in no way saying the people at the church are perfect, but it's the amazing acceptance and them letting me know that I can reach out if I need to; that makes the world of difference. The respect in my decision to not drag anyone else down into my family drama is there, and just go to focus on video production to escape the troubles of my family has not been an issue at the internship once; and I've been interning there for almost five months now.

That's the amazing thing about finding a community or great support during difficult times. You get so wrapped up on spending quality time with great people that for a moment the difficult situation fades out of existence and you find peace. You enjoy the time you spend with your support, in any given group of people. It could be among friends, family or coworkers; either way you'll know when you're stress about one situation fades while you are excited to spend time with a group of individuals who are just there to have a good time. And having the group be there for you, makes it priceless.

If you are going through such a rough and traumatic time and you don't have friends, family or a community to go to for support; I urge you, dear reader, to look for a group or community. What are you interested in or passionate about? Are there any local groups or communities that have a club or option to be a part of a community with them? Keep expectations low for the community and focus on your interest or passion, in time that will do the work in building relationships with the group where you're all just going to enjoy the passion and help each other build skill. If you're unsure of an interest or passion, try something new; you just may find a passion or surprise yourself with a new skill.

Sally Taylor

Chapter Seventeen

mass destruction in your own mind. Deconstruction.

Response: "I'm not comfortable because I'm not interested in that kind of relationship or trust in someone…"

"Cat's outta' the bag," here; yes, I'm asexual. I don't find interest in sexual encounters, instead I love discussions that focus on the deep truths of people. I'm not entirely sure why I've taken the path of not interested in romantic relations but I can piece together many pieces of this puzzle to find a very rough idea. Some main puzzle pieces are my own difficulty in trusting, my insecurity in saying or acting bad and turning someone away, my fear that it just won't work out and hyper aware of the current divorce rate; thank you parents for making that fear more of a reality scare for me. I see my odds are massively stacked against me, I'm afraid to even try because what would be the point? If you're statistically doomed to fail why even try?

I think a main reason for those defeating questions that I tend to have ruling my thoughts is that I've been let down too many times as a child. I have so much hope in someone and it all didn't end well. It's not saying anything bad about the other person, in these situations the fault is mine. I tend to place high expectations on people when I start expecting something. Many times, the high expectations are impossible for anyone to reach, even my own self. I see it now as a self-sabotaging manner that I don't always consciously have awareness of. It's something that I've taken time to pay more attention to and not have as high expectations but it's a process that will take time, patience and practice to unlearn this behavior.

How does asexual tie into all this? It's fear of not being good enough for someone because, in the past, it was incredibly difficult just to keep hold of friendships. I learned to not trust and not let anyone get to know me. Fear is the driving force in this matter.

The best past situation I can use is when I lost the relationship of a best friend. When I was in pre-school, I met an individual that turned into an instant friendship. We hung out together so much that many people questioned if we were actually sisters. Our friendship grew quickly and then when we reached second grade, based on where we lived in town, we had to attend different schools. From second grade through fifth grade, we were still amazing friends that just attended different schools. Then in sixth grade, we attended the same school. Middle school was particularly rough for me. But I was thrilled to have my best friend going to the same school again.

Just like any relationship or friendship, people change over time. And my best friend made new friends at the other school and kept those friendships at the school in sixth grade. It was great because I got to meet new people and build friendships. But like my friend, I had changed too. With school particularly rough, I was struggling to keep grades up and even attend school. I didn't build social skills like most students so I didn't understand social norms like I should have. Instead, I was living in terror trying to protect myself and just survive. Home life with family was difficult, school was terrifying to go to because I had certain bullies that really had a field day with me. I'm not trying to give excuses, just showing my perspective.

In seventh grade I was able to go on a field trip, it was long distance to Tennessee and the school rented travel buses for parents and students to ride to Tennessee. The trip was fine until heading home. We stopped to eat dinner before making the final drive home and I was sitting at a table with my friends. My best friend was sitting by me and we were all joking and having a good time. I didn't notice that my best friend may have been dealing with something but her mood changed so quickly.

That situation of having fun with friends changed quickly to my friend trying to suffocate by choking me.

I was crushed. I fled the table when I could and sat with my mom who didn't see any reason to figure out what was going on or if anything actually happened. I felt very isolated and alone and was going through a very traumatic experience where I felt I could talk to no one because no one cared.

That ended the friendship since pre-school instantaneously. I avoided this friend at school for then on. I didn't feel safe. I don't think that one incident led to my struggle to trust or let people get to know me, but it definitely played a key role. I refuse to let myself communicate to people to let them know me because I'm afraid after I open up no one will want to stay and I'd be let down and isolated again. I have the defeating idea that I can't take another hit like that but in reality, I can. I just don't want to go through that pain again because it hurts and it's not fun.

Here's the thing, nothing is worth it if not a challenge to fight for. If it's easy to accomplish then everyone could and it's not that great, if it's something truly worth it then there has to be work put into it to get it. Then you'd appreciate the accomplishment of all that work led to this great thing, person, or situation. No one ever says life will be easy, but if you know how to put the work in; it will pay off.

Because Trauma…

Chapter Eighteen

The very fabric of your wellbeing, your self-esteem.

Response: "I don't have enough trust to open up to someone on this…"

Tying in with the last point, trust. I have such a difficult time trusting people. I've tried trusting in the past and it didn't work out. Either I was backstabbed or it was the wrong person to trust. It's a struggle to trust when I communicate and someone's not interested or caring enough to actually hear me. I don't appreciate being treated as if I don't know anything, many times I do and if not, I'll try to brainstorm with the person to still try for a solution. If I'm truly out of any ideas, I'll say I don't know. When my own voice or opinion is not valued, I'm stuck there silent thinking about a solution and not understanding why no one cares to know a solution rather than fret over the problem. When I struggle to trust, I'll not put effort in speaking up; you can figure it out for yourself…or not.

An example is working on a group project in school. If each student has a specific role in the project and I try to communicate my part to the group yet that is not taken seriously, ignored or even interpreted wrong (to an extreme), and the project doesn't have a great outcome as what it would have if I was heard; I'm not particularly a happy camper because our grades were all affected in a negative way and I'm a student that tends to take school very seriously. I'm a very dedicated student. One semester I drove 7 hours for a project, another I slept a couple of hours in the back of my SUV to make a meet time for a project and it was below freezing that night. When I woke in the morning, the outside of my vehicle was completely frosted over.

I'm currently wrestling with the emotional pain of not trusting my own mother. Too many times she's told me one thing but either changed her mind and didn't update me or never meant what she said in the first place, after many years of this my trust in her has faded to the point of not trusting anymore. Not to mention trying to communicate to her something important to me and her either ignoring or not hearing what I say. A very real example is making a decision on some books at her home, there was a duplicate copy of a book in a series and I was taking the series to my apartment and was asking what to do with the one duplicate copy. I let my mother make the decision and then I repeated what she said to make sure I heard correctly and that she understood the discussion.

Not even 24 hours later she was asking why I didn't take the book from the series, and it definitely triggered me. Even having her make the decision and me repeating back her decision does nothing in having her actually hear me or be a part of a conversation with me. This isn't an isolated incident; it's happened over and over for many years.

To say I've given up on my own family hearing me is an understatement. I've noticed myself limiting what I communicate and it's to the point that my own family doesn't really know me anymore. I've picked up new interests and skills that my own family has no awareness of and it's challenging to spend any time with them or just talking with them because they're relying on old information that's not relevant, and I can't update them because I've already got it set in my own head that they won't hear me. I'm believing there's no point in wasting my breath, it will lead nowhere. I've not only given up but I've shut down on what's important or relevant to me now.

It's not easy to shut down from your family. I care so much but it feels like the relationship is too far one sided. On one hand, I listen and really hear when they have something to say; yet I don't get the same respect. And since I've distanced myself from my family I'm now not as connected or a part of the family and am missing out on important family events, such as the birth of my sister's daughter i.e., my niece. At the same time, I'm going on adventures that's taking me 7 hours away to another state and my own family didn't know that I drove 7 hours until months after the event. It was my own decision to not let them know because it was for a school project that I specifically reserved a ticket for and nothing my family would say could change my mind in going and I really didn't want to hear their criticism or judgement because it was doing something, I am very passionate about. The many months later when my mother did find out she did criticize and was very judgmental on how stupid I was even though it went fine and I got back with them none the wiser, I still got lectured. And at the time, I was 30 years old, fully capable of making those decisions and going out to take that adventure.

    I wish I had great advice on how to trust people but even now I'm still struggling with that and trying to figure out how. At this point it's built into my very nature and is going to take so much work on myself to break that habit that I naturally do without even thinking about. It's a process that I suspect will take many years but I hope to one day overcome my trust issues.

Sally Taylor

Chapter Nineteen

Don't fall for it. Never easy,

don't listen to your own mind,

Response: "I don't have the right words to explain this, why even try...?"

I'm a very abstract person, I love talking about theoretical topics and possibilities rather than facts and statistics. The way I communicate is based on concepts rather than details, when I'm speaking with someone who needs details rather than abstract concepts, the individual needing details is not going to appreciate getting concepts and will have trouble following along. It's not saying anything bad about someone needing details, I actually wish I was better with details and admire anyone who is great with details.

Along with being abstract and focused on concepts, I love to have time to myself to think about future possibilities. I love to 'daydream' of better futures or better ways of doing something. I'm very much a person that keeps to themselves and loves that quality alone time. I do tend to not speak much. And when I do, I'm usually speaking very abstractly or focused on concepts and it takes time for me to pull the details. Honestly, I don't care to much for the details because concepts can be reused for similar situations and the details can all change in any situation. I know to some people that's disrespecting details, I get it. Details are great, they are not my strengths; I'd love to be great at it but concepts interest me so much more.

That's where, finding the right words to communicate becomes a challenge. When I'm stuck in my own head all day and always focused on abstract concepts, I don't pay enough attention to the details to be able to have the right details to communicate. I'm not using this as an excuse, I know it's something I need to work on and have been since last fall. It's just not going so great.

I truly believe going to school for media production forces me to work on it because you have to be hyper aware of what is in the frame of the camera screen, if something is not meant to be there or meant to be somewhere else, you have to know to move it for filming. Attention to detail is important in video production. On one hand it's a big no-no to have equipment that makes it in the shot, like a tripod bag. Also, having only props meant for the scene is important because having something that's not meant for the scene could potentially mislead viewers. In my first week of video production classes I was working in a group and our group did miss the light kit stand and it made its way in the shot. Ever since then I learned to keep all equipment not needed either behind the camera or outside the room used for filming. It's worked out since but I still have much to work on.

I'm also socially awkward. I'm always checking before I speak to assess whether it's socially acceptable to say something or if I'll upset or offend someone in saying something. Usually leading to me fading into the background of conversations and missing so many chances to chime in. I like to have my thoughts clearly thought out before I say anything, consider as many variables as I can to make sure I'm not going to say something I shouldn't. I'm getting another lesson in this very thing because I've found a passion through my video production classes and am very excited about the passion and want to communicate to the world my passion. It's a problem when you're wanting to communicate something and a group of people you regularly hang out with don't agree with your own passion.

Details are, individuals at an internship that I was a part of for the fall semester. It was a requirement for the senior class to have experience interning through a company outside the school in the required field that goes with the major. Mine being media production, a video production internship is what I needed to look for. I was hired at a church that adapted very well to the pandemic and started broadcasting videos of their services. That required a video production team and they were looking for interns.

It wouldn't be right to communicate a passion for all things paranormal at this church because the viewpoints clash and differ greatly. At first, I didn't say anything. I kept quiet and kept the paranormal on the down low at the internship. It was a challenge when I was attending four paranormal investigations to film for a class project and needed to block out dates of interning. I was asked why I needed the time off and had to give a little detail of going to paranormal investigations.

At first, there seemed to be interest; the other individuals seemed intrigued by what I was doing. I found out later that the beliefs still differed greatly. But it was too late. I was eager to talk about the investigations because I thought intrigued meant it was ok, when really it wasn't. At this point, I'm realizing and adjusting my communication to not talk about the paranormal because it's leading to disrespectful for the individuals at the church. And that's fine, if I'm interning at a church then I need to be fully focused and invested in the job at the church. This is just a time where my own social awareness and judgement on what's acceptable to talk about failed. It wasn't the right things to communicate, I was way off on what was an acceptable topic.

Because Trauma…

Chapter Twenty

Your own train of thought, sabotaging.

Don't listen to your own defeating,

Response: "Why does it matter? Why would anyone else care?"

Asking why it even matters or why someone would even care is a defeating question someone who's been through a very traumatic experience. People will usually say this to themselves because they feel broken down so much that they don't see why anyone would. I've communicated this to myself so many times. It's giving up on others and giving up on yourself.

It's not the approach to take, yet it's taken so often. Usually followed by someone's self-esteem being lowered to nothing and feeling like they don't matter enough for anyone else to care. Or taking a defensive approach of not asking for help because someone doesn't trust other's enough to allow for the help. Trust me, I've been in both situations. Neither are great.

I struggle greatly with low self-esteem. I've always just wandered around feeling like the worst person in the world and that I'm not worth it. Then I'd get mad when I was going through a traumatic experience and no-one was decent enough to step up and stop the horror. It was wrong of me to think that, trust me; I get it. After a while I stopped waiting for someone to step up and do the decent thing and instead defended myself. Then when someone did try to step up, I shot them down and refused the help. I'll admit, I was vengeful. I thought that if I wasn't going to have the help before then I step up and take charge myself, no-one has the right to help now because they failed me.

    It was very difficult to see this wrong in myself and I cringed when typing the paragraph because I see now how wrong it was, now. It's currently January 2021, and I'm challenging myself to take a different approach. Instead of relying on myself I'm trying to work past the trust issues and allow for someone to assist if that's what they want to do. Instead of approaching the situations as if I know how to resolve the problem or situations, allow someone else to teach me what they know. If someone offers, sure I may know but someone else may know a different solution that might actually work out better. Approach every minute, day, situation, encounter as if it's something completely new and allow whomever I'm with to teach me what they know on a solution instead of me communicating to them what I think I already know. My methods don't always work out best and maybe there's something I'm missing that another individual has already figured out.

My hope is it gives the spotlight to someone else to shine and show them that I do value and care for what they bring to the table, and maybe that would lead to building trust and this could lead to a more accepting nature in both myself and the other individual. Hopefully, leading to less stress and more corporation, to being productive and working together; it's overall a great outcome. I truly do value and care for what other's think and have to say, I've just fallen to the wrong mindset and stuck with defensive survival mode too long that I don't even think about what wrong I'm doing.

When you're holding onto so much past trauma, it's difficult to have that better mindset. It took a lot for me to accept that. Last year I was very focused on self-development and self-discovery. The first part of the year was researching to try to understand, the middle of the year was a trial-and-error period where I focused on testing theories, then the last few months I was at the conclusion that there was so much I was holding onto from my past that wasn't good or helpful and I needed to work through the storm before things would get better. I had to stop trying to outrun the emotions from my past I so desperately avoided and just allow them to happen and work through them.

Honestly, it was the most difficult emotional pain I had ever been through. It was bad enough to physically hurt and I was too afraid to talk to anyone about it because I knew how much it hurt and I didn't want to drag anyone else through that pain. I also knew it was my responsibility to work through, and trusted that if it did get so bad that I'd know to reach out and ask for help if I started getting too "life ending" with my thoughts. I stayed focused on the future, I had to work through this and it wouldn't be forever; I kept telling myself to keep an eye on the future outside the storm where you've worked past all this and things will get better, because they really will.

    That's what got me through the last few months of 2020. By January 6, I had made my way through most of the storm and let go of so much of the past traumatic experiences. I don't see them and bad situations that I never should have been through anymore, but tests and challenges that help teach me how to deal with these unfortunate situations. All, to be capable of teaching someone else that may find themselves in a similar situation, help them or prevent the situation from ever happening for someone else.

I'm not saying I've worked through everything and it's going to be smooth sailing from now on. Not even close, I know I'm going to go through many more challenges in life and I'm going to have a choice of learning to deal with it or fall back to that same mindset from the past, and not learn from it but hold onto it for many years before it all builds up to something horrible.

Worried that I'd have to go back through another storm like the end of 2020. It takes great emotional strength to not fall into that trap and I'm sure I'll mess up again and fall into that trap but my hope, is that I don't fail in that way as much as before, and by being more self-aware of things and trying to think of ways to deal with situations and not let my own self-defeating thoughts win, it's a great start to a better future.

    But isn't that the whole point to life, learn how to navigate it? Learn how to trust yourself and others. Be creative enough to go with the flow and work through whatever life throws at you. To be independent, yet welcome any assistance offered and learn from it. Not one person knows everything, there are so many different perspectives from other individuals in this world and someone just might have a better way to a solution than what you may have. Why not be curious to what their perspective is and if it works out better, then you've learned a new skill and can use it and even teach it to someone else in the future. That's the beauty in individuality and being open to new ideas and different perspectives.

Because Trauma…

Chapter Twenty-One

self-talk, of all the…

Not worth it's,

Response: "Too much too quickly, now I'm drowning…I need time to recover, and breathe…"

This is something I'm not proud of and it's something that I believe was so wrong. I haven't had the best luck with doctors. But it's not all on the wrong decisions of doctors, honestly; I was either too afraid or didn't yet understand how to communicate an issue for them to know. Regardless, giving an individual high doses of twelve medications is uncalled for. It was so much that my own self was lost to the drugs and what remained, was a zombie like being that couldn't feel anything when it came to emotions.

I could tell the medications negatively affected my ability to function, yet it was me against everyone else. And being an 11-year-old kid with parents who don't understand how normal a highly sensitive person actually is, I was broken and needed the medications to be fixed. It seemed like a bonus to my family when it was so much that I failed to show any real emotion. Yet my own mother was concerned that I stopped smiling and always locked myself away in my room. Yes, I could hardly function and when I'm drugged up so much that it strips me of all emotion, smiling is not a possibility.

I went along with it for years because I was told by doctors and my own family that I needed to take all the medications, and as a child not an adult; you listen to your doctors and your parents. After years of being in a zombie like state, I was meeting with a therapist who was asking about the medications I was on and the dosages I was prescribed. I rattled off 12 medications and their doses as if it were nothing. I had taken the medications long enough, and had been asked enough times; I had the list memorized.

This therapist stopped me when I gave a medication name and a dose and asked if I meant 4MG instead of 40MG. I responded naturally by saying no, I meant 40MG. This therapist was horrified and recited the diagnostic information of the medication and the typical doses prescribed for the medication leaving 4MG last because it's the very high dose amount and expressed how shocked she was that I was on 40MG because it's 10 times the high dose amount. I had a picture of the medication bottle on my phone, I always did this just in case I did forget one of the 12 medications and I pulled the picture up that included the dose for the medication. It was 40MG.

That was the start of a change for me. I started to question more about why I had to be on so many medications at such a high dose. Then started realizing how unacceptable it was to feel like such a zombie. I tried asking my current doctor about the issue with too many medications but to this doctor, I needed all the high-dose medications and it wasn't an option to be lowered and proceeded to recommend electro shock therapy as an addition. It sparked the idea for me to get a second opinion. That second opinion led to another doctor horrified like the therapist at the list of medications, who suggested that lowering many is a strongly recommended immediate action.

The second opinion led to me sticking with this doctor and many medications from the list of 12 were in the process of being lowered within a matter of months. Because of the type of medications and the dosage, it would be a long process to get me off many and lower all as much as necessary. I did get antsy after a couple of years and just refused to take them cold-turkey. Bad idea, I know, it led to me completely falling apart and rampaging into a full meltdown. I couldn't deal with the rush of emotions I was suddenly able to feel, let alone all the other brain altering effects of dropping so many medications at once, still at very high doses. I got back on track but it took a few months of high concern for my doctor and family who questioned me every day on if I had any suicidal thoughts or if they could leave me for a bit to continue their lives.

It took a while longer to understand and learn how to deal with so much emotions and I'm sure my family thought I was worse for much of the time rather than doing ok. I didn't get a chance to learn how to appropriately deal with emotions, was too far medicated right off the bat to have any chance and it was new territory for me. It took much trial and error on my end to figure out how to manage the rush of emotion I could suddenly feel. It overwhelmed me but not once did I think about returning to a zombie state by being overmedicated. Instead, I worked more at figuring out how to manage my emotions and when I had a family that didn't outwardly express theirs like I did, I was much worse rather than better.

The zombie like state seemed more normal for my family because I was not outwardly expressing in a way that my family didn't naturally do, and they didn't understand. That's the price of being highly sensitive with parents that keep their emotions to themselves. I raged at my family because I finally felt like I could function and think properly and was horrified and not understanding how they could be ok with some things that were hurtful to others. I didn't have the ability to manage my emotions and was very upset for anyone who was on the hurting end of the family drama.

It's been a couple of months since, and I'm more than back on track; I'm no longer in a zombie state and off so much medication that I didn't need. My doctor is impressed with my ability to go to school full time and take care of the responsibility of living on my own in an apartment. Honestly, it is great. I love the freedom of my own space and the ability to feel human, not like a zombie. I've also learned how to step back from being so invested in the family and raging at them when another was being treated poorly at the detriment of building another up. I've learned more how to manage my emotions and how to be much calmer, and collected, yet I know I still have a long way to go.

Because Trauma…

Chapter Twenty-Two

and I deserve it's—Say you're fine,

when you know you're not.

Response: "I'm so used to and great with focusing on everyone else, I'd rather take a backseat to help others and I'll get around to myself when I can…it's fine…"

I've run from my own problems and emotions for many years. One way I was able to accomplish this was to focus more on everyone else and not pay attention or care much about my own needs. It became my normal, how I went through each day for many years that it quickly became automatic or something I didn't need to think about to actually do.

It's been only recently where I realized I needed to change what has been so natural to me. I needed to start taking more care of myself and my needs if I was ever truly going to succeed independently in the future. The last few months of 2020 I decided to stop running from my past and face everything I was still harboring head on and deal with it to get through this storm of chaos I kept wrestling with. I can definitively say, the last few months of 2020 was the most emotional pain I'd ever been through and I was dead set on making it through this storm, towards something better.

The best way I can describe the emotional pain is from research I did of two psychology terms, just combining emotional agony with high functioning depression; high functioning agony. I didn't want to get up every morning and it took so much more than I thought I was capable of to drag myself out of bed. I stayed focused on my goal of working through the pain to something better, that it wasn't going to be forever and I just needed to get up and get through the day. I had responsibilities that I needed to keep up with or it would prolong my future plans for graduation and I was so thrilled that I was going to graduate with a bachelor's degree. If it meant reminding myself every minute of every day what I was trying to get to, just so I'd get up and keep going then I'd do that; and some days it did require that.

By January 6, 2021; I had understood and worked through so much that my own emotions fell into check and I felt like I could breathe again. I felt ok I felt like I was getting very close to being better than back on track. I was able to get up each morning and not drag myself out of bed but climb out ready to start my morning routine with a cup of coffee and a few good moments with my cat. Things weren't perfect and I still had much to work on but I could tell the significant improvement, and it felt great.

I didn't have a great start with focusing more on myself. I was in the middle of school and struggling with the family drama. I spent more time focusing on school because it was going well for me and when I wasn't, I was keeping to myself with quality alone time. I didn't reach out to my family to talk nor did I answer too many of their calls. They didn't call often either. It was early 2020, the pandemic just took a dramatic turn and campus quickly adapted to all online format. I couldn't go to campus to use the computers to get projects done and needed a useable computer. My step-dad suggested buying a new computer and the cost split three ways. My mom and stepdad's contribution would be an early graduation gift. On the drive to a nearby store still open for people to go shop to buy a computer capable of running the programs needed for the projects, my stepdad started in on how selfish I was being by focusing on school and myself.

Honestly, it shattered me. I hated my own self for not feeling like I was a part of the family but couldn't take the drama, I didn't need my stepdad to contribute. I knew it wasn't great, I was hating myself enough for it but was shaken up with how my family was ok with the drama that was hurting many in the family. I had to walk away and focus on school because the stress was negatively affecting me.

I tried to communicate and ask why the horrible damaging drama was ok but got nowhere. Having no energy left to be a part of it, I needed to focus on myself to continue on. The comments my stepdad gave were very hurtful and it really broke me. I wanted nothing more than to be a part of the family but when the drama is so bad that it's hurting so many, I want no part in that.

Everything doctors and other prominent individuals were saying is that each individual needs to practice self-care. That it's super important. And that's what I was trying to do and the result of that was having my stepdad criticize me and say that I'm being so selfish? How is anyone supposed to deal with that?

I didn't deal with it well. Unfortunately, I completely unraveled and unloaded on my stepdad, horrified and hurt I was triggered and immediately was defensive and started defending my perspective. It in turn, triggered my stepdad which led to a full argument. Leading to me begging him to just go home, the computer was not worth it and a complete mistake to split the cost three ways. He didn't and still continued to the store. And I shut down refusing to speak anymore.

There are so many things I could have done better. I wish I did but when someone's so worn down and emotionally destroyed by very hurtful family drama, triggered is the first reaction. It's instinctual at that point.

It's been over a year since that moment and I've tried working on self-care and not being so triggered by my unhappy family who thinks I'm being selfish by trying to take care of myself. My conversations with family are very limited. Unfortunately, things continued to get worse for months and I chose to walk away and accept that I'm not a part of the family anymore. My school schedule is very busy with being a full-time student and working an internship. I know I set up my busy schedule as a way of validation when I turn down family events, just as much as it's trying to make the most out of my last year before graduation.

I know there's so much wrong in my approach but I've tried communication and it failed quickly. The drama is just too much and I need space to breathe. I make the decision every day that I've walked away from my family and every day I struggle with hating myself for it. I'm afraid my family will never know the depth of hurt and self-hate I feel for this decision and how it's negatively affected not only me but the entire family. They are angry because I don't open up anymore but I've given up on trying. My hope is that this distance is not forever, that one day I can be a real part of the family again. Right now, it's not realistic and not a valid option for anyone.

I can't change my family nor could they change me. So, the decision to walk away and let them be who they want to be while I be who I want to be is the only way the hurt stops between us and we move on with hopes that time with space heals.

Because Trauma…

Chapter Twenty-Three

It's simple, here,

put on a facade.

Response: "What's so wrong with trying to make sure everyone else is ok and happy, is people pleasing such a bad thing? No, I'm fine, these aren't negative coping strategies or self-sabotage, who cares anyways; I'm dealing with some serious crap..."

I'm really starting to be hyper aware of trying to please others at the detriment of myself. So, people pleasing. I'd rather make sure everyone else is ok and happy then I'd worry about myself later. I'm still trying to understand the depths to this but what I know currently, is that I can pick up on when someone is unhappy very quickly. If in a group and someone is not agreeing to something or getting unhappy; I'll go out of my way to help this other individual feel better, even if it means more work on myself. That's to make sure the peace is kept between everyone because if everyone else is happy then I can figure out my own need for being happy later and I don't have to pick up on someone else's unhappiness at that time to add to it.

Another way of thinking about this is a very recent example I found myself in. I got up early one June morning during 2020 when the pandemic had shut down the world. It had rained the night before but I still wanted to go out on a hike in the local nature preserve, through the wooded trails. I started on my hike and quickly noticed the rain from the night before was going to be an added challenge to the hike because the trails were muddy and some even flooded. I should have turned back and waited for a better day but I charged on through the woods making my way down a very steep hill.

The scenery was stunning and my focus was on all around me and not at my own footing down the muddy trail. I tripped and twisted my ankle, going down hard on my knees and one elbow. I heard a very bad cracking noise from my foot and it brought me back to sixth grade when I had twisted my foot in a similar way and had to walk from one end of the school to the other to make it to the nurses and later finding out from a doctor that I had walked on a broken foot. It took time, but I was able to get up. The pain was not good. I was concerned but knew I was a mile into the woods and checked my phone to see no cell service. I had two options, either make my own way out of the woods or sit and wait for who knows how long for someone to show up, and I ask for assistance.

I first checked my knees and elbow. My elbow had blood running down my arm, it wasn't terrible; just really scraped up. I could feel my pants sticking to my knees from something wet, sure enough they were really scraped up too. I tried walking and could feel the sharp shooting pain from my foot. I knew I had a long way to walk so I tried gritting through the pain and push on. There was a point where I realized it wasn't sprained but it was actually broken. That was when my foot swelled to four times the normal size, the cracking didn't stop but continued with each step, and could feel bone in my foot moving in a way that it's not supposed to. It was shifting during every step and the shift was not normal. The pain was just like sixth grade only in sixth grade I clung to the lockers, half dragging myself to the other end of the building; I don't have lockers or walls to do so, so the pain was so much worse.

    I refused to call for assistance or go to the hospital to get medical treatment. My thinking was that it's the middle of the worst in the pandemic for 2020 and the hospitals are swamped with enough individuals who really need it and I can manage with my foot, it's not life threatening or that serious. I didn't notify my family but instead went home, iced and wrapped my foot for a month while staying off it as much as possible. I didn't need to add more upset from them and I already knew I made a stupid decision and didn't need them to criticize and add to how stupid I felt. I understood that I made a bad decision and I was paying for it with a broken foot. It takes nothing to make a simple call when I reached cell service and ask for assistance, but it took so much to do so and knowingly create more problems for someone else; when I truly believed I could figure it out on my own. With all that being said, it was very stupid of me to not say anything and manage with a broken foot. It took longer to heal and even months after I still noticed some lingering effects that was evident, I had made a very bad decision.

With traumatic experiences, sometimes someone would rather stay silent and deal with it themselves rather than burden someone else and stir up trouble for them. It can greatly be from low self-worth or low self-esteem, or their own critical standard of needing to be competent enough to figure it out on their own and be able to deal with things like that on their own. Which is true, but only at a certain extent. It may also be from someone who tends to be more of a people pleaser, who'd rather than find the right help for themselves; would try to manage on their own, even when the problem is far out of their league. There's no real logic to this, it's just emotions twisting into false logic that's making the decisions.

Chapter Twenty-Four

Say you're ok.

Hide it. Fight it.

Response: "I'm not sure if I'm making the best decisions, it's life; no one knows and just figures it out as they go, same goes for me…"

I'm far from perfect. In fact, I've made so many mistakes. I have no idea what I'm doing and I'm pretty much making it all up as I go. In more recent years I took a serious turn from my typical to knuckle down and get serious about self-development. That resulted in months of deep research, many podcasts of motivational speakers on repeat, my own trial and error tests, and figuring out what wasn't working and what to change to try again until something worked.

I had made not so great decisions during this time because I didn't know and I was frustrated feeling like I couldn't turn to my family. I was very ambitious at times and took on too much and failed miserably. I went through the moments where my family was struggling to keep up with the changes I was making and they lashed out because it was too much too quickly. There were many heated conversations between me and my family, usually leading to both parties feeling incredibly hurt and frustrated. There are so many things that I could have not said or said in a much better way, the same goes for my family on the receiving end.

I've been hurt by some choices certain family members have made and I first started with trying to communicate that this is not ok and to find an alternative way of going about that. One family member in particular, continues to choose not to hear me and make the same hurtful decisions. I reached a point of complete frustration where I'm already on edge knowing I'm about to be around or communicate with this person. That's no way to start because it's set the entire situation up to fail. It's not right for this family member, I get that. I have no patience left or hope left that this person will actually hear me and make alternate decisions when I say that's hurtful don't do that again. It's so much more difficult when I try to forgive this person but this person refuses to take any accountability and instead would throw anyone else under the bus just to avoid saying I messed up and I'm sorry. There's no closure or moving past this now because I don't know how to forgive someone who can't acknowledge or take accountability and just apologize and try not to make that mistake again.

I'm not trying to justify on my behalf with this, just trying to provide perspective. I know my approach so many times were very wrong. It was out of triggered hurt emotions and not thinking in a logical way. With that being said, it wasn't ok; and if Karma is a thing, I've paid for the wrong things I've said.

I love my family. More than they will ever get. I tried to communicate to my family how much but could get that message through to them. One example that led to the worst ending was when I couldn't take sticking to the sidelines of the family drama that I now call "the great family divide." Something between a cousin and my sister left the family divided and ready to attack the family that wasn't agreeing. I don't know the full story of what led to this but I did try to find that understanding. I failed miserably. I went and just let my cousin talk and give as much of her perspective she wanted, making clear that I wasn't out to push blame because I didn't care; I just wanted the family to reach a resolution and blaming isn't the way. It was a great thought but one person was able to turn that completely against me.

I was calling my mother after a stressful day at school and was wanting to ask about starting to get another perspective on the family drama, and was hoping for some advice; she answered and proceeded to tell me how much of a burden and inconvenience I am to the family. That's a blow that's going to continue to destroy me for years to come. And I did not take it well during the phone conversation. I proceeded to unravel and lash out saying that I worked so hard to find a way to resolve this family drama and school has been rough and all I wanted was a little advice. The phone conversation ended with me hanging up on her because I was hurting so much. That evening I got a call from my sister who was six months pregnant.

Our mother had called my sister and gave a very fabricated story to her, who was stressed enough and didn't need more while being six months pregnant. My sister then decides to call me and completely scream my ear off. I was horrified that our mother would have the nerve to stress my sister out more by this during the challenging time she was going through with the pregnancy, and that she also gave my sister a version of this story that is "fake news," because it was so far off-track and not what I had said.

I had to take those twenty minutes of my sister screaming in my ear before I could get one word out myself. The first thing I asked was where she got this information because I was counting all the inaccurate information in what she was screaming to try to figure out what was going on or where it went so wrong. She told me that our mother had called and told her and I tried asking questions to try to find a starting point of giving what I actually communicated versus the fake news our mother fabricated. My sister refused to accept anything I said and instead said that I had betrayed her as a sister. It didn't take long before I had to accept that I wasn't going to get the correct information through and I had to let her hate me and just get off the phone. My hope was that I'd be able to repair the damage between us but it's been almost two years and the relationship between my sister and I is non-existent.

It kills me every day knowing that if the fake news our mother so happily decided to relay to my sister had not actually been given, and the conversation was kept between my mother and me; which I've made very clear early on specifically because I knew my sister didn't need the extra stress, I'd still have something of a relationship with my sister. And I've tried to ask my mother to apologize or at least acknowledge giving the fake news to my sister so I could begin the process of forgiving, yet she's chosen to respond by saying she's not taking accountability for anything.

Me not saying anything certainly could have helped in having a relationship with my sister as well, and saying that I was triggered and destroyed by the comment right from the start of being a burden and inconvenience is no excuse. I should have just hung up that moment rather than let my hurt emotions call the shots. But there I was, hearing someone I care so much for tell me how much of a piece of crap I was. And it still hurts. And sometimes there are some statements you can't come back from, they just do too much damage that leads to destroying not only the person but the entire relationship; maybe on a level that can't be undone, fixed or to recover from.

I believe that no one really knows what is best during a traumatic experience, especially when it's a situation you've never faced before. And you can either let the experience defeat you or you can figure it out as you go and do the best you can with what you have. There will be choices that turn out to be more of a mistake but that typically would be realized after the fact and during it may have appeared the best decision just on a get through it or even survival basis. Sometimes emotions are running high and they cloud the ability to think through the situation before responding. If you do respond by your emotions, remember that there's no logical basis behind them. That doesn't mean they are wrong or invalid, they are what make you human and are a necessary part to existence and knowing when something isn't right. But after that, it's best to step back and wait to be able to think it through and let logic step up so you can make better decisions.

Easier said than done, trust me I know; it's something I'm still trying to get myself to remember to do before reacting by my emotions calling the shots. I have a long way to go but I can say that acknowledging this and making a point to work on it is the first step in the right direction. With time, practice, and a little patience with yourself; it can be done. I wish you nothing but the best in accomplishing that. There really is something to taking a moment to walk away and think or process before going back and dealing with the situation.

Because Trauma…

Chapter Twenty-Five

Ignore it. Bury it.

Conceal it. Heal it.

Response: "Why waste my time trying to communicate? I won't be heard…"

I don't talk much. I'm either in my own world of thoughts or too much of an introvert to speak up. When I do, it's because I put enough thought into what I need to say and I tend to not talk about some random useless bit of information. There's meaning and a purpose behind what I say. When I finally find my voice and try to communicate, it's a tough blow when family doesn't hear me or tunes out what I've said. It makes me second guess at saying anything. I've done that a lot lately. And now, my concern is the family doesn't even know me anymore because I've chosen to not speak up. I have given up because of my thought process of if I've not been heard before why try wasting energy to be heard again, when the pattern shows it's not likely to happen. I have a lot of traumas surrounding the feeling of having no voice. The year 2019 was especially difficult not just because of the pandemic but because my grandmother passed away and she's the only family I knew that actually heard me and would look into it and try to do something, if there was something wrong.

    I grew up in terror. I'm not trying to exaggerate here, there's real terror for a child who doesn't understand why one of their parents turns into a monster and would hit and hurt, and going to the other parent did nothing to stop the pain and terror. No matter how many times I cried to my mom of being hurt and not feeling safe at home, it did nothing to stop the pain. I had to learn to accept that this was going to continue, I couldn't rely on anyone to stop it even if I was too small and young to myself; I had to just endure and live like I was always walking on eggshells. If years of this doesn't do traumatic damage, I'm surprised whoever went through the damage; is still alive. It's not easy and there's real psychological damage from years of that. Twenty years later I'm questioning my mother as to why it was too much for her, to hear her kids cry out in pain. And every time she tries to invalidate, say it never happened, or push blame on someone else. All I really want is for her to acknowledge, take responsibility and give a real apology; but for whatever reason, she doesn't.

    I can tell that I'm giving up on my mother again. I don't talk to her much now. She truly doesn't know me anymore and I know it's because I won't talk to her. But I've given up. I'm destroyed by her invalidation tactics and her unwillingness to take accountability for me to begin to forgive. That's all I want is for her to own up to the mistakes so we both can move on to something better. I need closure.

Instead, I'm not answering her calls, deciding to not spend any time with her, and not opening up to her on what matters to me so she'd have a chance to get to know me. My last birthday she gave some decorative pillows of a movie I loved but she didn't know that I lost the interest in the movie over a year ago because, she wasn't a real part of my life. It hurt because it only proved the damage done by not feeling like it was worth communicating to her anymore thus, not communicating about anything that mattered.

I think self-esteem, self-confidence, self-worth and hope all ties into someone not wanting to speak up. When so much in someone is destroyed that they feel so low and give up hope that communicating, it's difficult to find anything that would help. Many times, someone just finds a way to make it on their own because of the belief that you can't rely on anyone else, that they'll just let you down or stab you in the back is so great that going through the horror on their own seems better. Relying on your own self to figure it out seems better than taking a chance at someone else hurting, is far better than taking that chance to reach out when reaching out really is necessary. It's something I'm still trying to work through, my destroyed relationship with my mother clearly shows that. I'm not on speaking terms and I don't see how I will ever be again. It's something so upsetting to me but I don't know why I should try to talk if the message will not be received by her. To me, there's no point.

I know I'm wrong and I'm sure there's a way to communicate where she'll actually hear me but, I feel I've tried so much and failed and don't have the hope or energy to try what little options I have left. I'm also struggling to find any more options. One of the most damaging guilts I'm going to have to live with and struggle through every day now is knowing I've given up on my family. It will haunt me for the rest of my life, but I lost all hope and failed so much.

The best idea I have left is to pick up what shattered pieces of my life still remains and find my own path away from my family knowing that I've given up and failed miserably on them. What hope I have left is hope that I'm trying to save for a day, where years from now I could return to my family and things would be ok. But even then, that hope weavers constantly because I've fought for my family for so long and was completely destroyed by it. Hope really isn't much of a promising option for me now.

Chapter Twenty-Six

You know you can't.

That's not how this works,

Response: "I'm not great with sticking with my values, I know it's an uncertainty for others…it's not fake, it's adapting…"

I'm more interested in making sure the peace is kept between others. I can adapt very well with different groups of individuals as well as enjoy, appreciate and respect their values, beliefs, interests, etc. There are boundaries, I'm not so interested in being a part of a group that has the intent to do harm to another. I value respect so much and any group of individuals that shows great respect is something that I'm going to love being a part of. With this natural ability to adapt, I can change my own interests sometimes on a dime. One group of individuals may be avid sports fans and another avid gamers, I may not have a high interest in sports but enjoy spending time celebrating a win with the sports fans just like I don't know too much about gaming and am not great at it, I still love learning and playing a new game and appreciate the enjoyment of a fun chill game night.

Both the sports and gamer ideas are not the best representation of how well I can adapt. On one hand there could be an avid gamer who also loves sports. For me, I'm not very invested or interested in sports or games and when I'm not spending time with a specific group, I'm not likely to spend time watching sports or playing many games. Currently, I have high interest in my future and where I'm going with it, so I'm more likely spending time working on my future plans. Then when I go spend time with a group of individuals interested in sports, I'll enjoy focusing on sports because it's more important to me to have the great connection and quality time with the group of people.

Having this natural ability tends to cause problems sometimes. Many individuals who notice this, spark concerns and have questions about me being fake. I understand where they get this concern, it can be very alarming to have someone change course with different people so effortlessly. It's difficult to see where I stand on things, adapting to the tone of vastly different groups and having a good time and connection with both can be jarring for some.

For me, I don't care quite as much about the styles or tones of groups but care about the good quality time. If everyone is happy and being respectful of one another then I'll have a nice time connecting. I think it has to do with conceptualizing the connection and all the other details like interests, beliefs, etc.; can all change to work with keeping the concept of having a really good connection with some good people.

    I understand not everyone can view friendships or connections in this way. It's not saying I have a better advantage or anything; in all honesty, I admire people who are sturdier in their values, beliefs, and interests. There's this vibe of having much more figured out and being able to stand on their own in their values and beliefs where I would tend to jump around to many different ones to appreciate and learn a little about as many as I can.

Sally Taylor

Chapter Twenty-Seven

it's haunting…how your past,

always finds a way,

Response: "Yes, it's controversial, I get it. I'm also my own worst critic…"

Something that greatly frustrates me about myself is how I battle my own doubts on things I question with making sense or not. The saying, "You are your own worst critic," was meant for individuals like me. I've had a number of classes where I would have a conference with my professor to be critiqued on my work and I'd easily out critique my professor. They'd end up telling me to go easier on myself that my work wasn't that bad. I'd be gung-ho trashing my hard work where my professor would go much easier and just be asking for minor fixes.

Everything I work on will always be trash in my opinion. It doesn't meet my standards of good or acceptable so I'm more than ready to completely trash it. Yes, it's obsessing on having the work perfect and never reaching perfection. Perfection is an idea that doesn't actually exist. I know this, yet I still push myself and trash my own work because I still struggle to see my own work as good enough.

It's even more challenging when I have a professor so excited for my work saying it's so great that I shouldn't try to "fix" it anymore and just "leave it alone." My thought process is, "Sure, it's good now; but I can figure out something to make it great or even better."

I don't know how to respond or how to leave my work alone when I have a professor saying it's great and to leave it alone. I disagree because in my perspective there's something that could be improved. Since no one will ever reach that perfection level, there's always going to be room to improve. So why not make it better, why leave it at just good? This is something I've lost much sleep over by fretting about and working myself up so much on a project.

It may also be my very low self-esteem or self-worth where I believe I'll never be good enough or do something good enough. I want to be able to do something that I'm needed for because I'm amazing at it. I want to be useful, yet feel I'm completely useless and a failure often. The catch is, realizing this feeling will never go away and to not give into it. Just keep working and doing my best but also giving myself time to relax and not obsess over projects. No one's going to reach perfection and not everything will be an amazing and great piece of work, it's doing your best and putting effort into it that truly counts. Showing that you know how to and even showing that you're working for improvement, even if its small steps; they matter. That's definitely worth something and more times than not, it's enough.

I struggled through grade school. I didn't like it and it wasn't because of the academics. Grade school students can be very immature, and I grew up in grade school just before bullying was really focused on as an issue. I skipped often in middle school I learned how to ask for the bathroom pass early in class and spend the class period hiding in the bathroom and when I returned, I gave the excuse of a bloody nose that wouldn't stop. It only works so many times before teachers start getting suspicious so finding more excuses was a necessity. It's not something I was proud of; I just couldn't take the bullying. I ended up dropping out of school in eighth grade which scared my parents and led them to find a private school for me to attend. It was an hour and a half ride on a bus to the private school every day, one way.

This school took academics in a very different approach. There was no homework and the teachers taught for five to fifteen minutes before saying, "Ok, do whatever you want now just don't kill each other," then the teacher would sit at their desk reading a magazine or something. Students could listen to music at any time during the classes, they could play games on their computers they brought and snack at any time during class. After about a year of this, I figured out how much I actually liked and needed homework.

I started almost begging my teachers to give me homework. I wasn't being challenged and it frustrated me because I loved learning something new. I wasn't dealing with the horrible bully situation so I was able to relax a little more and appreciate the ability to learn. Yet I was only learning foul language from hearing other students instead of learning anything that would be important. I failed at having the teachers give homework and after a year and a half I was done and wanting to risk going back to school in my hometown, just to get homework. But it was more than just homework, I wanted to learn, I needed to be challenged.

It took another year and a half before I convinced the superintendent of my hometown school district that it was time to return to my hometown school. By then I was a junior in high school. The first week was just getting re-accustomed to the demands of the public school system only it was high school not middle school. Also, learning to re-acquaint myself with my old classmates that I was unable to stay and deal with because of bullying. To return to three and a half years later was another challenge I needed to prove to the administration at the school because it seemed like they were waiting for me to fail, to be able to send me back to the private school.

I kept my head down and didn't draw too much attention to myself and that worked because I navigated in a public high school with little bullying issues and ended up having enough credits to graduate as a junior grad. The feeling of not good enough really spiraled into its own being then. I jumped straight into college and felt like the most underprepared college student. I felt like I didn't belong because in my mind, I still only had an eighth-grade education. I attended the public high school for one semester and I knew it wasn't enough to make up for the three and a half years of learning nothing but foul language. I couldn't shake the feeling of being so far behind. And it was a struggle getting my associates.

The feeling of being so far behind didn't leave me until my second year going for my bachelors that was more than ten years after I graduated high school. Even then, I still had lingering questions of whether I truly was intelligent enough to get my bachelor's degree or if I still was an imposter. The hard work and my grades helped to combat those defeating thoughts, because I excelled and thrived.

I'm afraid I'll always battle with these feelings of not being good enough because that's just how I am. I push myself to be better and set standards that's impossible to reach because I want to keep trying for better. It's how I learn and how I improve. It's just knowing the fine line of pushing yourself too far that shouldn't be crossed. And I've learned, and I still need to remember to, occasionally set time to be laxer with myself and give myself permission to step back and not let the work be perfect. No professor would say I'm not dedicated or a student that bullshits their work. I've had a number of projects where I put so much more effort, time, and energy into what it was actually worth. A few projects took me out of state and countless hours up all-night editing footage. I'm a very dedicated student that takes the homework and school projects seriously. It's something I'm very proud of and has taken years to finally shine through.

Because Trauma…

Chapter Twenty-Eight

to find you, hunt you,

catch up to you, blind you,

Response: "I know this sounds crazy, why speak up to sound crazy; I'll just stay silent and not give the chance to be seen as crazy…I'm dumbfounded by this actually being a thing too…"

One of the most challenging things I've struggled with and am still struggling though is knowing when something sounds crazy yet is so real and I can't say anything because no-one would hear me and take it seriously.

Early on, I've struggled with my parents believing I'm so mentally messed up that nothing I say holds value or should be taken seriously. It's a brutally lonely life because I've long since shut down on really communicating anything because when I try to, I'm not heard.

I have so much I've learned and so many more questions yet I can't communicate or ask because it's too weird for my own family to take me seriously or actually hear me. I've given up on trying to communicate and what's resulted in that is my own family doesn't really know me.

The best example is my interest in a movie, I used to like the movie Nightmare Before Christmas enough to have shirts, blankets, stuffed animals and many other assorted things that was from the movie. A few years ago, my interest in the movie ended and I wanted nothing more to do with the movie, I had another interest that took its place. A few months ago, on my last birthday my mom made me pillows with the characters from The Nightmare Before Christmas. It broke my heart because she still believed I was interested in the movie. I hadn't been for years and it resembled for me, how much she wasn't a part of my life and didn't actually know me.

This wasn't all on my mother, I chose to shut down more because I gave up on trying to communicate. I'm too hurt by not being heard that I've decided not to even try to speak up. I'm trying to protect myself by alienating myself from the very people I care about. It's not something that works, I know this; I just haven't figured out a better solution yet.

I'm not seen as a very logical person because I protect my own sense of logic from the world. I guard it because I value it so much and fear it being hurt or disrespected. I'm seen as very emotional and for many, you can't be emotional and logical, it's one or the other. And since it's not my job or not high importance to try to change the views of people who only see me as emotional to where they see and even value the logic, I hold so close; I don't really show my ability to be very logical. That's a side of me that I continue to hide and protect.

It's easy because I'm more focused on other's and how everyone is doing that, I filter my way of communicating to adapt to not upsetting other's, even when being brutally honest is a better path in the long run; I still filter to please. It's because I struggle greatly with stirring up conflict. I'm very sensitive to conflict so much so that I'll do what I can to prevent or stop conflict, even if it's to the detriment of myself, even if it adds more challenge or work to myself. It's not something that really works or is a smart plan to always do but I struggle greatly with conflict. It's something I still need to learn a better way of navigating and knowing that some conflict or tension is ok, it's how some individuals learn and figure out something isn't working.

Because Trauma…

Chapter Twenty-Nine

keep you guessing,

panicking,

Response: "I can't think about it, it freaks me out too much…"

I avoid my own emotions and problems, that's the gist of it. I do this because I'm scared to deal with it all. I fear that I don't know how to or I'll not like the solution that I'd rather avoid my emotions rather than deal with them. I'm super critical of myself and I don't have great experience in dealing with my emotions. Though I'm capable of being very sensitive or emotional, it's a struggle that I'm not great at dealing with. I should be, but I'm not.

Typically, if something traumatic happens; I go in a mindset of shut down and do what I can to get out or away. I stop engaging or communicating and just function to get out of the situation. Later, I tend to drive for hours, go on a long hike or deal with it by ranting alone in my own space. After I've ranted and got everything out of my system, I don't want to chat more on it. It's difficult because I've had situations where other's pried for me to talk about it and that's typically when I explode with emotion and just unload.

Sure, that's great to process through with another person but it's just as traumatic to do that than it is going through the situation prior. I carry traumatic events with me but as long as I'm busy staying focused on things I need to do, I'm fine and not thinking or dealing with the emotions from the traumatic event. Sure, it builds up and it's not great to have the idea to just always stay busy; but I'm not quite at that place to be able to talk and not let talking be just as traumatic as the situation.

Another concern is when someone is so hurt that they have trouble trusting just anyone. I know this situation all too well. I've had medical professionals try for over eight years to get me to open up and I struggled to because I had such a difficult time trusting them. Sure, I understood they were here to help and I needed to let them do their job; that means nothing when you've been through something that greatly damages your ability to trust. An even more challenging situation is when you finally try to trust and you give more information and it ends up backfiring or being a mistake. When someone has trust issues and takes a risk, having it backfire on them really damages the chances of taking another risk.

I feel for anyone experiencing trust issues, I've struggled with this most of my life and the ironic thing is I give people the benefit of the doubt more times than I should and think much better of people than I should. I'm very optimistic and tend to view people in a much better light and then I give a little trust in them and completely feel destroyed by it later because I either gave too much trust or chose the wrong person to trust in. I've noticed in the past few years my desire to be more connected in the world and take more risk but I've also noticed my hesitation and fear in opening up increase. That's the strange paradox I'm currently dealing with. I'm sure I'm not alone in this. It's a challenge, but not impossible to navigate.

    If I'm being honest, my communication skills or my decision to open up more has now decreased; yes, I want to be more connected with people and engage more but I'd rather enjoy the moment with them and listen to other's open up rather than open up myself. The unfortunate thing, that's not how relationships or friendships work; there's a give and take on both sides and in order to make more of a connection, being open is required on both parties. I'm scared to open up again. I'm not doing well emotionally and my world seems to have fallen apart. I'm struggling greatly and failing miserably. My trust has been damaged so much that I'm ready to be one of those off-the-grid hermits in the woods that keeps to themselves and has no other human contact. At this point, I don't know what else to do and the emotional pain is at an all-time high. I know I need to just take time and the pain will pass.

Finding another perspective and finding a way to give a little more faith in people is the only starting solution I've come up with, and it's hard; especially when you feel so beat down and unable to trust. And yes, it's a starting point; because it's going to take more than a little work. There's so much change in myself that I need to make and its grueling tedious work. A long journey that may or may not play out well. The only real way of knowing is by trying and putting the effort in until you see positive change or a continued downfall.

The point is not to keep offering trust to have destroyed, it's to find the right people to surround yourself with that you can trust and work on building your own capability of trusting by giving a little faith in those people. If you're around the right individuals, they'll hang around to help build you up rather than betray your trust. I found a group of people, more so a community; through interning for my senior portfolio, I worked on a video production team at a church that took advantage of broadcasting their services for individuals to still be able to attend church, at home. They reached out to my campus asking for interns and offered to work with the campus and student if it was for the student's senior portfolio class requirement. I had been trying for an internship for over a year and was losing hope in finding one, when I came across this opportunity I applied and felt like it was going to work out, it was more a gut feeling.

I landed the internship and it technically was over the first week of December but I was asked what my thoughts were for hanging around more. It was such a great fit with the individuals I worked with that I loved the idea. I made a personal decision, going now outside of the school; to continue an internship going through the church. Another semester has passed and I'm still there interning and appreciating every great moment with the individuals I work with.

I found the individuals who would not take advantage of someone offering trust. I know I'm much more damaged than they realize and I bring to much baggage for them, I keep my personal traumatic experiences to myself and just enjoy the time I have interning there; if anyone were to directly ask, I'd consider my words and what I'd give before communicating it. But it's not something they are responsible for, it's something I have to work through. I'm much more hopeful that I can work through all this just for being a part of this video production team, even if I leave my baggage at the door.

It's possible to find good people to put trust in. I didn't believe it before but this church community showed me how wrong I was. And, if I can, anyone can.

Because Trauma…

Chapter Thirty

fearful.

Will you ever be whole?

Response: "I can't focus on my limitations or I'll never attempt to surpass them…"

Call it the rebel in me, I'm not particular crazy for someone to tell me what I can and can't do. Many family members have tried and in response, I did what I was told I couldn't anyways. For me, I see that as a limitation and I don't like to have limitations established on me. I'm someone who has defied odds on a regular basis. My limitations greatly differ in myself and are not the same as everyone else's. In fact, everyone has their own personalized set of limitations that may or may not be similar to another individuals. Just because you can't, doesn't mean I can't. I'm referring to completely legal and ethical situations, like sports for example. I'm not talking about crimes or something as horrific as having the ability to commit murder or something.

One of my own examples, I signed up for a unique activity that would take me states away from Illinois to the state of Iowa. I had family members tell me before I reserved a ticket for this activity that I couldn't make that drive. It dumbfounded me. I had my own car, I scheduled the time, I had the gas money, I had the funding for the event, I had the route planned out; yes, I'm able to make this event. Instead of arguing with my family who told me I couldn't, I stopped talking about the whole topic and event and still reserved a ticket. I got up early on the day of, all packed and ready to go; and I took off for Iowa. I made it to Iowa safely, attended the overnight event and made my way home the next morning. It was months after when my family learned that I had actually made the trip.

I've personally had so many people try to establish limitations for myself and it's frustrating because they are not actually my limitations. I want to do my best, push myself to be better; if I were to abide by what others deem my limitations, I'd never accomplish pushing myself to be better and actually get to anything better. I'd rather find what limitations I actually have by trying and decide if I want to push past it or if it's a limitation for a good reason to stay a limitation.

Take sports for example, you're in a race, running as fast as you can, you're so tired and ready to be done, you keep pushing yourself to run, your friend that's competing against you is gaining and passing you fast, this is a race where you win against your friend every time, yet their winning now. A limitation would be to accept that you can't beat your friend this time, not defying the odds or finding a second wind or pushing yourself enough to run a little faster and manage a win. Your body was telling you that you had no more, yet, it is so much better than giving up and accepting a loss. Managing to find that drive to kick into faster gear just enough to pass your friend and win. Despite the pain in your legs and feet screaming at you to stop, despite your heart-rate skyrocketing and the feeling of not being able to inhale and breathe. That limitation was by far not a brick wall but an obstacle you can overcome and succeed while setting the bar for a new limitation.

So, how do these examples play into traumatic events? How does this concept align with traumatic events? Quite well actually. Going through a traumatic event is tough, and many people deal with or don't deal with traumatic events differently. Some may go on a run to process through their emotions, some may journal, some may push the event out of their mind to not deal with it; regardless of the method chosen after a traumatic event, not one method works for everyone and sometimes individuals think another individual who's been through a traumatic event needs more or less assistance in processing or dealing with the event, and pressure or don't pressure the individual enough to help them through.

An example of this, the 9-11 attacks in 2001. All of America seemed to fall to pieces, for a valid reason; the terrorist attacks were horrific and very traumatic. All I knew to do at the time was try to assist my sixth-grade classmates to the administration office so they could call home or lend an ear to cry to and be supportive, I don't think I managed to process the event for months because I couldn't ignore the panic and pain of my classmates. I was fine with that, assisting my classmates was actually very therapeutic.

What I struggled with more was having therapists that were pressuring me to open up more and fall apart over the event. I didn't understand why I was expected to fall apart over something that I had already found my way of dealing with and being ok. It may sound insensitive of me, trust me; I cried over the event just like everyone else. I just found my way to cope quickly by focusing on the panic and pain of my classmates and the drive to make it just a little better, for them in whatever small way I could.

Another example, for not getting enough support on such a traumatic event. A tricky situation that may be from the individual not speaking up or some other reason that makes it not intentional to not have the support but the impact of the traumatic event or the event itself is not known. If it is known, and there's still a lack of support; it can be defeating to be so hurt and seeking support but everywhere you turn for support it's massively unhelpful. Probably the most disappointing moment to feel so alone in this traumatic event and it's not an event horrific enough to be worthy of finding support. In this case, you're irrational and crazy to be dealing with this…which is so false and wrong in so many ways. You went through a traumatic event and need to find someone to assist in processing through or dealing with it, that's incredibly rough and I'm so sorry to say that the other individual truly won't understand your pain because they are not you and they didn't go through what you went through. The need to process and deal with the aftermath is still valid and very important, don't diminish your pain because you can't find anyone that understands. All I can say is keep searching for someone who can assist in processing and dealing with such an event and don't give up on the search.

Because Trauma…

Chapter Thirty-One

Will you ever make it

out of this…

Response: "I can't discuss this; I need my pride…"

It's incredibly difficult to talk about a traumatic event because many individuals feel like they are weak for bringing it up and feel it's better to deal with it alone in silence rather than be seen as weak. There was a time where I believed that had lived that mindset. My own past traumatic experiences festered alone in my head and ended up causing much more trouble years down the line. I also learned how wrong I was to believe that I needed to keep it to myself, it's not weak; as a matter of fact, it shows great strength to be able to bring it up to talk about and find a solution from somewhere or someone other than yourself. Others can relate and may even have a great perspective to a solution, you may even have the ability to assist someone else or prevent a traumatic experience for someone else by speaking up.

Pride is such an unusual concept. It holds the power to prevent someone from speaking and also holds the power to be an uplifting force in someone's life. Yet, with such unimaginable abilities; pride is still a concept, and not something you can physically touch, see or measure with your own senses. It's something many are very protective of and would hold their ground on defending.

But I get it. Pride is a difficult topic; it happens to the best of us and will continue to be a concern if we all willingly idle by letting our own pride dictate our silence on certain situations. Pride is not to be mistaken as confidence, self-worth or self-esteem. You could have the least amount of confidence imaginable and still be prideful. You can have the worst image of yourself and still be protective of your pride. Your self-esteem can be as low as the gutter and still stay silent because you don't want to damage your pride by speaking up. The same for having great confidence, great self-worth and self-esteem. It just differs, maybe, because individuals having so much of their lives put together have made their way through traumatic events and don't continue to let those past events control their daily lives. It takes time, but everyone has the capability of reaching that.

Sally Taylor

Chapter Thirty-Two

dark tunnel of life.

With no light to guide,

Response: "This is my problem; my responsibility and I need to figure it out myself…"

The idea of it's my problem and needs to be my solution, directly lines up with not wanting to be too much of a burden to anyone else. Also taking accountability and being able to be independent and work problems out on my own.

This might have spiraled out of control due to my difficulty in trusting others, not everything has to be figured out solely alone. People are sociable creatures; we were designed that way, and need to reach out to inquire from other's a different perspective to a problem or a little assistance in solving a problem. It's not always bad to reach out and ask, it becomes a problem when you do it too often instead of trying to work it out yourself first. If you rely too much on others instead of trying then it's more of an undriven and even laziness concern.

I remember a time where I leaned more towards just going to ask someone to assist, just because it was convenient. I started questioning why I was reaching out and was critical of myself, asking if I truly thought I needed the assistance and if I could actually solve it on my own. The answer usually, would clearly show that I wasn't so interested in solving it myself but taking a convenient route of asking another to assist.

I tried challenging myself to not be so quick to reach out and sit with the problem a bit to see if brainstorming a solution would lead to problem solved. Take car trouble for example, a great reason to reach out for family or friends to assist in giving a ride to somewhere so that you can get your vehicle fixed, you could also call a cab or an uber and a tow truck if that would be necessary. It's much more expensive but in these cases if you have a close relative or friend that doesn't mind giving a ride, be sure to thank them and offer to pay for gas and maybe lunch or dinner.

Something that wouldn't be a great reason to reach out would be if you are too tired to run to the store to buy basic essentials, or a pandemic hits, and you're too afraid to walk into the store. In this case, you have your own vehicle and you're just trying to find someone to do the very basic essential shopping that you just got to get over and go to the store. Listen to headphones in the store if that helps, grit though it because everyone in that store and all the stores down the road are gritting through it too.

Because Trauma...

I've also had many people, including medical professionals, tell me that I don't open up and talk much. I saw doctors and therapists for eight years and they all struggled to get something out of me. I am very guarded in what I say or what I talk about and it's because I'm very protective when it comes to traumatic events. I'd rather shut down and not say a word and dismiss it as "not a problem" while I internally spiral and work myself in a frenzy trying to figure out a solution. What finally got me to open up was my poetry professor.

I take my classes very seriously and put so much effort into getting good grades. After second grade I gave up on any future endeavor with poetry, I believed I didn't have a talent nor would I ever understand it enough to be able to write a good poem. And here I was in college taking a college level poetry class. I was terrified. I knew the professor from a previous class that was just a creative writing class, not specifically poetry. I felt optimistic that I'd survive the poetry class because this professor was very good with students, he taught by clarifying anything students didn't understand. I started the poetry class by appealing to a general emotion, leaving all personal experiences out I focused on a topic most of the world knows and can understand.

After the third poem my professor pulled me aside and questioned my reasoning for not using something that I personally resonate with. I was very upfront with this professor and told him my hesitations and fears of adding more personal topics and he challenged me to try saying the class would not end well if I don't because appealing to a general emotion is not what poetry is about. For my fourth poetry assignment I focused on a moment in my past where I was surrounded by grief and I was unable to feel grief myself and felt out of place. I turned in the assignment and waited in such a panic, I spilled every emotion from that moment and feared that I failed the poem.

    Instead of my professor validating the fear of failing the poem, he was ecstatic. The poem was exactly what he was asking for and was so thrilled that I was able to intertwine so much emotion in just a few stanzas. I took over the job of challenging myself by pressuring myself to go deeper and add more real moments full of emotion. Throughout the rest of the semester my poetry got deeper and expressed much more challenging emotions. Half way through the semester I decided to show some of my poetry to my doctor and therapist. Both of them saying that they finally feel like they know something after more than eight years of trying to get me to open up.

    Opening up is still a challenge, I still notice during difficult and stressful times I tend to lean more towards shutting down and not speaking up and I still have a therapist holding me accountable for that by commenting on my usual methods of getting very quiet and preference of dealing with it alone. It's been the first instinct for so long that it's like an automatic response that I don't always realize I'm doing until I've been silent for hours…or days. Breaking this habit is the new challenge that I'm still trying to figure out how to do.

An excuse or reason I tell myself for not opening up is that it's something difficult and upsetting, and I'd rather not drag someone else down by bringing it up. I always had the thought process of, I need to figure this out to not drag someone else down because I don't want to ruin someone's day by bringing up my issues. It's all my emotions and a situation that I dealt with or went through and other's that didn't don't need to experience that upset or pain. It's like I'm trying to protect others from this pain that I'm struggling with by continuing to struggle in silence while telling everyone that everything's ok.

The unfortunate realization is that it doesn't work that way. You have some very intelligent and caring individuals that just know when things are not ok, some may be good friends and some may be family. They know and if their highly sensitive or empathic, they still feel it. Saying everything's ok doesn't help, it just distances yourself from some really great individuals; who are hurt that you don't feel comfortable enough to open up and instead, toss out a lie that everything's fine.

If you're in too deep then you're in too deep. Don't chalk everything up as fine when you've got others around you trying to get you to open up so they can be there to lift your spirits. It's those individuals you need to lean on an appreciate for being in your life, because they do care and will work with you in trying to find a way to make life and situations better for you.

Because Trauma…

Chapter Thirty-Three

and no guide to light,

your way through this

Response: "I'd rather not say anything to not upset anyone and keep the peace, I don't want my struggle to hurt anyone else…"

Directly lining up with my last point, I'd rather not hurt anyone else by bringing up my issues and keep the peace or keep everyone happy. It doesn't work that way because most likely, you're acting strange or hurt and they already know. If they're empathic or highly sensitive, they already feel it too.

There could also be a situation where you'd have to call someone out who played a negative role in a traumatic situation and instead of being so ready and open to calling them out, for any reason you may find it better to just not say anything and keep the peace. Trust me, your thought process can find just about any reasoning to not speaking up, no matter how logical or bizarre that reason is; it can be very convincing.

Maybe someone is telling you to keep quiet at the risk of getting yourself or someone you care about hurt. Maybe you're afraid of what others will think when you speak up and fear negative judgement placed on yourself in doing so. Maybe you're overwhelmed by the situation and there's a long process to bringing it to the right individuals' attention to do something and you're too drained, upset and maybe even destroyed by it all and just want to forget and move on. Whatever the reason, it can be convincing.

But what if this is happening to someone else? What if you could be the very individual that helps so many more by speaking up? What if speaking up has the potential to not only save your life but the lives of others? I'm not trying to diminish the situation here or tell you that you have to speak up, just don't let fear be your driving factor in staying silent. If it's that much of a negative situation, then do it for yourself; if no one else at all. Find your way to get your life back to where it needs to be, it's not anyone else's right to hold that much negative power over you in that way.

Yes, it's going to hurt, not just be difficult for yourself; but you're calling some negative individuals out and they're not going to be happy. Don't focus on their unhappiness, instead focus on your own happiness and if others are going through the same situation, focus on their relief and happiness that the situation is over. Sounds great and everything, but it's not easy. It won't be all sunshine and roses when you're stepping up for your own life, but in the long run; it's worth it. It's a small moment in the concept of time that has started long before you and will continue long after, this moment will pass and another will start; just go for another path, and do your best at navigating away from such negative situations. Life is not so much a science but an art. There's no one right or wrong answer it just takes a little navigation to find the right picture. Believe in yourself.

Because Trauma…

Chapter Thirty-Four

seemingly ever endless

darkness.

Response: "I am world class at lying to myself. Talking about it forces me to focus on the truth of the matter, it makes it more real. I lie to myself and ignore it because I can't take the extra emotional pain…"

I call it being world class at lying to myself. Mainly because my own fear drives me to avoid talking about past traumatic situations because I'm afraid of how real it can get and how much worse the emotions can get. I'm afraid it will be too much and I won't be able to deal with my own emotions. I'm afraid I'll give up and see no reason to continue in this life. I'm also afraid I'll spiral into such a mood that I turn into such a horrible person and there'd be no hope for me. It's so much easier to lie to myself and not deal with the emotions of the past traumatic situations that just get buried, but here's the thing, they keep building up to so much more.

There may be some defensive mindset where I fall into this shock, just keep going with the mundane and ignore the traumatic event that just happened. I notice my own pattern of dealing with difficult and traumatic situations, it's been a thing for me so many times that I can't not take notice. (Yes, a double negative there.) I have a more recent example that represents how I deal with difficult and traumatic events. It's when I tried going camping between semesters, I attempted this on a very low budget and all on my own.

    I had my vehicle packed with a cooler, tent, and my camera; which I planned to go to camp at a place where I could be in nature and enjoy taking pictures for a couple of days. I needed to go off into nature to get away from the normalcy of town-living life. I was dealing with a lot of stress and a mini-vacation in the woods at a campground seemed like a great idea to feel better and recharged for the next semester. I found a campsite that was four hours away that worked with my budget and the scenery for camping was perfect for taking my camera and having a chill camping trip where I could take scenic photos.

    I drove those four hours, using my phone to google map me the directions. When I reached about 1000 feet away from my destination, that's when my concern hit. I was in the center of a busy bustling town, no-where close to anything related to camping. I pulled over and checked the address again, found the mistake posted on the internet and retyped the address to the campsite. The new address led me another three hours in another direction, not towards home, yet not away from home. Stressed and frustrated, I followed the directions again when I really should have just gone home.

After another two hours I was in another part of the state, not the state I live in either, and was getting concerned. I was taking backroads and in the middle of what seemed like nowhere. I thought it was a good sign and I'd really be camping and be able to destress and recharge for the next semester. Yet, I wasn't sure, and my concern and anxiety kept increasing by the mile. I reached 2000 feet away when I had to make one more turn down a road that I could tell, wasn't going to lead to a campsite. There was one sign I saw driving that "hinted" at camping but it was obvious that it was some sketchy attempt to convince people that there was camping where there wasn't. That was about two miles before I had to make the last turn down this, now dark and secluded road.

I turned down the road, continuing with the google maps directions and reached the point where my phone told me I reached my destination. I stopped and looked around, the road continued and there were no turn-offs to anything. Just road and hill on both sides. Less than 500 feet back I passed someone's home, a small rundown makeshift trailer that had a very loud dog in a fenced in front yard. Some ducks wandered around aimlessly and didn't seem bothered to wander right into the road to stop and squawk.

Because Trauma…

This was not a campsite; it was a posting of a campsite where some creepy individual could lure people to go camp and it would likely end horribly for those people. They'd likely not be seen again by their family or friends, not alive at least. I drove a short distance further to find a place to turn around on the side of the road to get away from the area quickly. The ducks had found their way to the road to stop, sit and squawk; not wanting to move when I drove up to leave. I creeped by and weaved around the ducks that seemed so much like an alarm system with the amount of squawking they were doing; and once I passed the ducks, I sped up quickly in a panic; so terrified that someone would be there stopping me.

I had a little less than four hours to drive to get home. I was stressed, scared, and was unable to process what I just avoided. Deep down I knew, and I knew it was also a narrow escape. Even now, I can't bring up some of the details of what surrounded me when I made it to this road that led to me frantically escaping. I could tell, it wasn't a place for people to camp but a place for unsuspecting people to disappear. I drove home in silence. I kept checking my rear-view every few miles to see if I did manage to have someone tailing me from that false campsite but after an hour, I had no concerns of being followed.

A full day, where I drove to find a campsite that led to me bolting trying to escape something very dangerous; ended up with me sitting up all night in horror.

I said nothing, I just drove home and sat on my couch all night, unable to go to sleep or do anything. The sun rose and I was still sitting on the couch in shock. Tears were running down my face. I was exhausted, up all night; horrified of the situations yet relieved that the situation didn't play out and it was a very narrow miss for me.

Sometime that morning I spoke with my mom on the phone. It was a difficult talk because I was unable to really say anything. I managed to let her know that camping didn't work out and it was actually a horrible situation that I narrowly missed. She was relieved that I made it home and wasn't hurt, I got off the phone and sat there a few more moments trying to figure out how to get myself to either get some sleep or get up and do something.

A few weeks later I was with my mom riding in the car and she commented on some family going camping and was extending the offer to me. The horror struck me so quickly and I told her that I'm likely not going to want to go camping again. This from the perspective of a kid that grew up going to family campouts. I grew up running around at campsites with cousins, aunts, uncles and grandparents just loving the time camping with my extended family. To not want to go camping again, for the next 20 to 60 years is quite a strong response. I stand by that to this day, and it's been a full year since I failed at camping. The attempt and where it led me, really got to me and deterred me from going on future camping trips; even with my family.

When I hear family comment on camping or ask me to go camping with them, I experience flashbacks of when I was frantically escaping that road with the squawking ducks and other concerning things scattered around that I'm still unable to speak of. My thoughts spiral into what could have been if I hadn't made my way home and spiral into who else tried to go camping and wasn't as lucky to get away as me. My chest gets tight, I panic though I'm able to know how to not create a scene over this, I still panic.

To not be in such a panic-filled mess, I push everything related to the situation aside, I don't think about it. I don't process the emotions I buried from that situation. I quit communicating when people around me comment on camping, instead I silently panic and look for a way to leave the conversation. I shove the topic and all the emotion from it aside again to not deal with it and continue my day. I'm avoiding my emotions that I buried, just to not deal with them.

Talking about camping, the failed camping attempt, or the emotions I have over those topics is something I'm not ready or open to do. I'm afraid that if I do, the realization of the situation would hit me and it would feel so much more real on how dangerous the situation was and how much I narrowly escaped.

I know some day I'll have to work through this past event. I know I'm not dealing with a more recent traumatic event well and it's going to continue as a problem until I work through it and get to a better emotional place. I will, someday; but I'm not ready to today and probably won't be tomorrow. It's not high up on the priority list of working through traumatic situations. But, one day it will be and I'll deal with it then.

Because Trauma…

Chapter Thirty-Five

It's defining.

Pulling you, down, down,

Response: "I feel bad enough, I see that I've failed. I don't need to focus more and feel even worse."

I know when I've messed up or failed. I beat myself up about it all on my own. I don't need any external forces or people to contribute more of how much I've failed at something. Talking about it is the right thing to do as far as owning up to the mistake but continuing to harp on it to almost drill it in my head isn't necessary, that creates more of a problem rather than gets to a solution. I am my own worst critic, and I hold true to that so well. If there was something that I messed up on or it hindered or affected someone in a wrong way; I'll know and already be holding myself accountable long before anyone has a chance to bring it up.

I'm the same way with my own work in class. Which is the best example I have. I've had so many professors who required students to turn work in to be critiqued and would get feedback on what to work on to resubmit and try for a better grade. Those professors quickly learned that I'm able to completely trash my entire project by saying everything that's wrong with it and different options to make it better. The professors would have to tell me to stop and that my own project wasn't that bad and just to work on a few key points for an A.

I'd still struggle with that because I'm someone who fully believes that something can always be improved in some way and nothing ever gets to perfect. It may get to the point of good enough but not perfect. Call me a perfectionist or call me someone who likes to push myself for my best, it's likely true for both and I'm not likely to stop soon. Even if you've reached the best in one aspect of something, there's still room for some improvement somewhere else.

I'm world-class when it comes to beating yourself up over something you've messed up on, as well. I take it to the extreme like trashing my work better than my professors ever would. It doesn't matter if it's something minor or major, I'm still my own worst critic. I'm still trying to understand why and the best understanding I have is that it had negatively hindered or affected someone else, and when I'm so driven to be helpful or useful; achieving the opposite is brutal.

I will spend hours running what went wrong through my head and what I could have done better, attacking my own decisions as "so wrong" and it would loop over and over until I've found the best way that I could have done it for future reference. I destroyed my own logic and trashed everything I did to make sure I remember not to mess up so badly again. Having another individual chime in and tell me how bad I did is not going to make me realize anymore or learn any better, trust me; my own brutal accountability has been taking care of it for the past several hours. If anything, I'll not deal with another individual speaking up and would feel attacked, probably because I've been attacking myself for the past few hours and having someone step in to beat it even more to the ground causes more harm than good.

If you throw the scenario of a traumatic event into the mix, don't you think the person at the brunt of the traumatic event has been through enough? Sure, a mistake may have led to a traumatic event, but the whole situation of the event is enough for them to realize where everything went wrong. If they're clearly struggling with the ramifications from the traumatic event, it's not the best idea to drill them about the mistake but rather approach with compassion and empathy and see if they are ok and not in need of assistance. Otherwise, they may see fit to give up in life and think the best solution is suicide. Maybe that's what this world needs more of compassion and empathy.

I know it's hard to lead with compassion and empathy, trust me; I've struggled to lead with both as well. When you're more of an awkward introverted person, having surface level conversations all the time is likely the most unappealing interaction and I've avoided talking to others as much as possible to avoid getting pulled into some random conversation. It's where I've messed up in life, because it leads to being an outcast or feeling alone all the time. I've only recently tried making a change and being ok with random surface level conversations. It takes time and work but with enough practice there will be improvement. I've seen it in myself.

Chapter Thirty-Six

deeper. Into this abyss.

Struggling to breathe,

Response: "I've built up too much from trying to outrun, why can't I just continue to ignore and not focus on it. Things always get tougher before better and there's too much I've been outrunning, I'm afraid I don't have any chance…"

It becomes a problem when you've ignored or repressed emotions from a traumatic event, and when you've done this time and time again; that's a lot of charged emotions that you've built up. Over time, it gets harder to deal with them when you're ready to work through it all instead of continue to avoid and repress. I took that path, it's not a great path. I refused to deal with difficult situations and emotions for years and it all piled up and no one could get me to open up for the longest time. I was so great at keeping it all to myself and I'd shut down and close myself off from everyone, it led to me isolating myself so much so that I alienated myself from everyone.

When I finally decided to deal with everything from my past, I had gathered so much hurt emotions that it almost seemed like an explosion of emotion. I was lashing out and hating the world. I knew what was going on, I knew I was wrong in lashing out yet I couldn't stop myself. It was just too much. I continued isolating myself and exploding on people so quickly and I kept hating myself for being such a terrible person. News flash, that isn't the best idea when you're trying to work through past traumatic experiences, it almost defeats the purpose because you can't be harsh and hate yourself while you're trying to work on getting yourself better.

I struggled to deal with the fact that my own emotions are my responsibility. It took me so many years to understand and accept that. I used to get upset about something and it would take nothing for everyone to know about it. I didn't care to be responsible with my own emotions mainly because I didn't learn to do so and struggled with feeling like such a zombie because I was on so many medications that it hindered my ability to function and have any emotion. It's still not an excuse, I could have stepped up and done better. After the majority of the medications were gone, I felt such a rush of emotion return and I didn't know how to deal with it. I lashed out and was a terrible person. It took me being aware that I was acting poorly and making the conscious decision to do better.

It's been a long journey and I'm nowhere close to having my emotions in check, but I've made serious progress. I still see myself falling back into the same patterns of shutting down during very stressful and even traumatic situations and it's tough for someone to get me to open up. It's what I'm so used to doing that breaking that natural habit takes time and a lot of practice.

Even now, I'm struggling with a situation in my family where I'm trying not to shut down and manage my emotions better but I'm failing at it. I'm also navigating the problem of hating myself because I feel like I'm being so selfish when I should just be happy for the family member involved. I spent about an hour with another family member and noticed my own failing spiral into silent tears and short close-ended responses to her questions. I wasn't hiding the fact that I was hurting and very unhappy, and it bothered me greatly. I knew better and didn't understand why I couldn't pull myself together to enjoy the short time I spent with her.

The situation was I got word that my sister is expecting her second child. My mind spiraled into all the hurt emotions from her last pregnancy and how upset I still was over being excluded and the damage from that leading to having no relationship with my sister. It kills me every day knowing that our relationship is basically considered non-existent. After many attempts to work on a resolution with my sister and being shot down each time, my hopes for reaching a resolution was dashed and I gave up trying. It breaks my heart but if she doesn't want to work through things to repair the damaged relationship then there's nothing I can do. I have to walk away, broken hearted and defeated.

I took the path that doesn't work out or lead to anything good. I avoided my own past and tried out-running it for so many years and the emotions tied to all that I was out-running had built up. To move forward you must work through the storm of emotions and when you've out-run that storm for so long letting it rage and build, you've got a serious storm to work through and it's going to be so much more difficult. I was always afraid to deal with my own emotions and didn't know how to even begin to deal with them.

The best advice I have is to not try to out-run past traumatic events and the emotions that follow with it. I'm just afraid that this advice is coming to you, reader, too late; because you are reading this looking for advice meaning you've already made the decisions you knew to make that may not have been the best option. It's not your fault, it's just life. You do what you think is best and sometimes it doesn't work out as well as you'd hope. I commend your effort. Now try again but by doing something different.

Because Trauma…

Chapter Thirty-Seven

there's one way,

swim harder,

Response: "I've set up so many defenses and barriers, I'm afraid to tear them down and let someone in; I'm also unsure of how to tear down defenses I've had for many years, how do you break such a habit or defense?"

I grew up building walls and barriers to hide from difficult situations and keep others at a distance from fear of negative judgement, and the desire to hide such tragic events as to protect others from that pain. I know how difficult it is and if I can mask it enough so no one has to deal with it too, that would be great.

When someone spends much of their time for many years building walls to hide from the rest of the world, it becomes difficult to know what walls need to come down and opening up is more of a challenge than an easy solution. It's like a natural response that's automatic, to establish walls that hide the world from the storms. Or, would it be to hide inside the walls from the world? I'm not sure anymore…

More recently, I confided in a friend at a place I was interning at. I was hurting and needed a little guidance and let myself open up on the family drama that had torn me up. I was wrestling with the idea of walking away from my sister and feeling like a horrible person for doing that. This friend gave the most respectful advice and I was able to take a few days to process and was at the point of deciding to walk away by the weekend. I was interning at a church, every weekend I'm attending all services to work on the video production team; so, the weekend message really gets through to me.

This weekend was no exception. It was the very kick in the rear I needed, the message resonated so well with the struggles I was having with my sister and family. There were a good number of times I was running switcher and during the pastor's message and would say ouch because there was a point the pastor hit that really nailed it for me. By the end of services, I was set on being ok with walking away from my sister.

When I was leaving the church, it was just after 12pm on Father's Day. I called my dad to check the plans, I thought I'd be spending the rest of the day with my dad and sister. I was prepared to grit though it but when I called dad, I found out how dramatic the plans turned. He told me he spoke with my sister that morning who said that she heard from our mom that I'm not going to be at any family functions that my sister is attending anymore. My head spun.

Every form of hurt, rage, depression and pain shot through me. I've had many conversations with my mom, numerous times, on how I was upset with how bad things were between my sister and me ended with my mom saying she was not going to say anything to my sister. She always responded by saying she was not going to get involved. The last time I spoke to her on this I did say I wasn't willing to attend another family event with my sister there, but all the context before that statement is key; I was saying I didn't know what more to do and I can't keep trying to reconnect and resolve things when I'm getting shut down at every attempt. I was out of options, I had to walk away; that was the only option left and from what I learned from the internship, that's ok. My mom again said she'd not get involved and that I was putting her in a difficult position; which I then commented out of pain that maybe she shouldn't have fed my sister the "BS" she fed her in the first place, then we'd actually have a relationship.

Normally, I'd call to question my mom on why she lied and why she'd "BS" with me again. In fact, that was every time before; that I'd call and completely unload. This time, it was different. This time, I'm holding to my boundaries that my mom so effortlessly steam-rolled over, I did not call but rather blocked her number and she now has the pleasure of me cutting complete ties and walking away in such an abrupt manner. I'm done. I told her many times that I can't take her "BS-ing" with me anymore. It was time I stood strong with that, my boundary was severely disrespected and cutting ties was the result. I have to take charge of my wellbeing and unfortunately, that meant having nothing more to do with my own mother and sister.

It's so hard to let go of any possible future relationship with a parent. It's like you lose a key piece of yourself when you cut those ties. The pain stems from all the hurt from the abuse all the years before and the hurt from accepting there'd likely never be a good relationship with the parent in any future. There's slight hope, that the abuse will finally be over and you can finally thrive as your own person; which masks only a tiny portion of the pain.

In the end, I knew this was inevitable. I knew I was biding my time with my mom and once I graduated with my Bachelor's Degree, I'd be taking off to start over. I was just planning to keep biding my time and not completely cut ties so soon. Sure, I have six months before graduation; but that's six months of pacing myself, on distancing myself from my mom. In hopes that it wouldn't be so abrupt for me. I guess it was time for plans to change, time for an abrasive abrupt end to a relationship. Thus, here I am, in my apartment, sitting on my couch, typing this chapter, in full water-works tears; because this hurts so bad. But, it's ok, this was necessary; I will recover and be ok. It's just going to take some time.

Maybe I'm finally barricading walls that my mom will never get through again, maybe I'm not. Maybe some walls are good and necessary, and they are those healthy walls that are more boundaries rather than barricades to go into full protection mode where no one hurtful can reach you. Maybe for some people, it takes a complete barricade. And maybe it's ok, you are not such a horrible person for barricading someone out after they've steamrolled over your boundaries time and time again. Now all you need to do is take time for yourself, focus on self-care and recover. Let time do its job and heal.

Because Trauma…

Chapter Thirty-Eight

for that surface,

keep fighting…

Response: "I've been dealing with this alone for a while, why should I let anyone else in to help now?"

I've been hiding an aspect of myself from the internship ever since I started interning at the church. It has to do with my past and the negative side effects from it. When I was eleven years old my parents took me to see a psychiatrist. They believed there was something so wrong with me mentally. This psychiatrist's own greed got ahead of him and he took advantage of my parent's concern. This psychiatrist decided to prescribe some medications, but it didn't end there. This psychiatrist kept increasing the dose and adding more medications. It led to being on twelve medications at extremely high doses.

What my parents were hoping for was this psychiatrist would help in getting me to function normally but what they got was a shell of a person that wasn't able to function at all. Every emotion, every bit of myself was stripped from me because I was so drugged. I was the very definition of a living zombie.

With a number of the medications, there was a side effect of Tardive Dyskinesia, which is an involuntary neurological movement disorder caused by drugs prescribed to treat certain psychiatric conditions. One medication, at a high risk of Tardive Dyskinesia, if taken for a long period of time is Haloperidol. I was told by a therapist that a very high dose of Haloperidol was 4mg. I was on 40mg. I had taken it for many years and started noticing the uncontrollable tremor movement in my hands and some subtle ticks in my face that were starting to increase in severity and frequency. It took time but with a new psychiatrist I was able to start to lower the Haloperidol, in hopes to get completely off. My panic and impatience got the best of me and, after a year of weaning twelve medications slowly to not spark serious medical effects from going cold turkey; I took that risk and just stopped cold turkey. It wasn't my smartest move but even now if I were able to go back in time to make the choice to continue the plan to wean off instead of jumping to cold turkey, I'd still make the same decision of cold turkey.

Much of the Tardive Dyskinesia has corrected itself but I still have some moments where my hands still shake and my face has moments of jerky ticks. My concern for going to school for Media Production was at an all-time high when I started interning for my senior class requirement. I was hired for an internship on a video production team where I'd have to run around backstage with a camera to film live shots. It gets incredibly difficult to keep a camera steady when your hands still have moments of a jerky shake from Tardive Dyskinesia.

It was my hope that I'd find a way to manage without having to bring it up to anyone at the internship. It was touch and go a few times, but I've been interning there for almost a year and still haven't mentioned my troubling past with Tardive Dyskinesia. Thanks to the pandemic, much of my time interning required me wearing a mask so the facial tics were masked when they were present; but the facial tics are not as prevalent as my hands jerking and shaking.

I figured I'd not said anything for almost a year, why would I bring it up now? I've managed this long wouldn't it be better to just continue as is, and not comment on dealing with Tardive Dyskinesia as I was running the camera. It would almost seem like that would be a situation that they'd be upset at me for not speaking up because, they could have found ways to combat the times where the camera was just too shaky and me knowing why and fighting an uncontrollable involuntary movement. Of course, I may also be overthinking this and it all may be fine and not an issue; I tend to do that, over-analyze things.

For the Tardive Dyskinesia situation, that is a traumatic experience mainly because of my long journey as a living zombie and all the side effects from being so drugged. Projecting my need to stay silent on the Tardive Dyskinesia is likely my way of avoiding my own pain and upset over the whole ordeal of years on so many medications at such high doses. I'd rather not bring up years from my past where I didn't even feel human. I'd rather forget and move on, and the idea I got from that was to not talk about it and pretend it never was and hopefully one day; I'll recover and be ok.

Nice idea, but it's really not realistic. It just doesn't work that way and I'm going to have to work through all the emotions I now have over those years where I didn't feel human, if I want to ever get past it. I'll get there, one traumatic experience at a time; I'll find my way through and finally be ok.

That's just one experience I've been through where the trauma has been so much that for any number of reasons, I'd prefer to deal alone and not let anyone in. It's mainly out of fear, hurt, and desperate desire for the trauma not to be real. Sometime, I prefer to deal with it alone because I don't want to be a burden to anyone else. There's also the situation of having trouble in knowing who to trust and instead of taking a chance at getting hurt again, I'd rather keep it to myself and just deal with it alone. Can anyone relate?

It doesn't matter what the reason for staying silent and dealing with it alone is, it's not something that would end well. It doesn't work. Eventually, the pain and turmoil build to the point where you can no longer contain it; and there's an explosion of emotion, an outburst, a meltdown. I've learned this the hard way and the unfortunate truth is, I still resort back to the same patterns of staying silent because it's something I'm so used to and something I've grown comfortable with.

It's much easier for me to shut myself off from everyone rather than communicate and let other's in to help with something I feel so out of my league on solving or healing from. Breaking this pattern of shutting down has become more of a challenge than anything and it's something I have to work at little by little, every day. All while knowing there will be days where I'll make progress and days where I'll have setbacks.

Because Trauma…

Chapter Thirty-Nine

…for your purpose.

You still have a chance,

Response: "These defenses helped me survive, do I really need to start tearing them down; what if I need them again, I'm not sure it's safe or best to tear them down."

It's now my understanding that I have a difficult relationship with fear. I think because I grew up in fear all the time, I'm stuck in survival mode. I struggle to trust anyone and everything I do, with making decisions and my own behavior and actions are all rooted out of fear. It's a difficult conclusion to get to; but when I think back, I can see how much fear has directed everything about me. I'm stuck in survival mode and because I've been in this way of being for many years, it's become my normal and I don't know how to break it. I see how it negatively affects my friendships, relationships and acquaintances.

Sometimes I'm aware of my fear directing the situation and still struggle to do anything different. My internal dialogue runs wild, beating myself up asking,

"Don't you see what's going on here? You're better than this, stop it! Why are you doing this, it's not ok." Yet I'm a passenger at this moment, watching myself act in a way that I know is not me. I let fear take the wheel and all I can do is watch as I spiral into an emotional wreck.

Maybe I've reached the first step in changing these old habits of letting fear take the wheel. Maybe in knowing that it's fear, I can find a way to combat it and not get lost in survival mode. I'm not saying this will be easy, no, in fact; it's going to be strenuous, draining work. I'll probably get frustrated at times and question why I'm even trying. I'll probably go through trial-and-error periods where there's more error than anything. But I do believe it's worth it.

I remember how challenging it was starting an internship. It was for my school as a requirement to intern somewhere related to the field I was studying. I was majoring in Media Production so interning with a video production team was the goal. I applied at a local church and right after the interview was asked if I could start by shadowing the booth that weekend. The first few weeks was difficult. I was overwhelmed with meeting so many new people and I remember sitting in the booth the first few weeks and when someone would get up to pass by behind me, I'd be so jumpy. I know others there noticed, and I was disheartened by my jumpy reaction.

No one ever said anything or questioned my jumpiness and it took a month or so before I stopped jumping and being skittish every time someone walked behind me. Truth was, I wasn't familiar with where I was or who the people were around me. I didn't know anyone and felt apprehensive to trust and didn't feel comfortable or safe. My feelings were wrong in that case because I was interning at a church that took advantage of video production during the pandemic, they are all good people; and I was just too uptight and unable to relax until I felt comfortable and safe.

I know I've made it this far with all the defenses I've set up. I was in survival mode, the best way I managed was setting up defenses. You either build walls to defend, get ready to fight or just freeze up. I wasn't the type of person to fight and freezing would have been much worse. The only option I knew of that was left was to build up my defenses to not let anyone in, to protect myself from everyone. And fear held the reins in this and went all out.

Maybe it's my fear talking now but I've spent the first part of my life building defenses, living in survival mode; I'm not too crazy about tearing down my defenses. If I tear down the defenses then wouldn't that mean I'm defenseless? I don't think I'm capable of taking on the world without my defenses. They work, why destroy them. Yeah, I get it; all fear talking. The problem with having so many defenses or measures to protect yourself from everyone is that you don't let anyone in to really get to know you. It's a very lonely path.

Because Trauma...

I say I want deep connections yet I keep people at a distance with a ten-foot pole. It doesn't work like that. It's a paradox I wrestle with daily. When I finally feel brave enough to take down some walls and open up, I'm timid in doing so and once I do; a real deep conversation happens. I walk away with a lot to process, yet feel so numb. That's just before the spiral. Fear steps up and creates chaos, panic over thinking I shared too much or I was wrong in communicating something and it makes me such a horrible person; this other person must think I'm a horrible person. It's a scramble to see if I can rebuild the walls, I tore down or if it's too late and I need to just hit the floor running and flee completely. Disappear.

It's much like when you corner a scared animal. They panic, shift into extreme survival mode to figure out do they need to run, do they need to attack, can they protect themselves? What needs to be done to escape and be safe? It's a bad analogy but it works for this idea. I don't know what the best approach is, I'm still trying to narrow down a good solution. I know my own way of living has corrupted my ability to make the best call on this. I know I'm frantically trying to correct some unnecessary habits. But how do you stop someone from living in survival mode when it's all they know to do? Not to mention the idea of Enneagram. Bring that into the mix, is this struggle to live differently hopeless or a lost cause? Yes, I've researched the Enneagram and Personality Theory, to try to understand.

I don't currently know much about Enneagram, but I'm jumping into more research. I had the understanding for years I was a five, now I see what went wrong in trying to work on self-development; I'm not a five, I'm a six. Individuals with enneagram six function from a fear base mindset. I'm hoping it's not too late for me, that I haven't let fear direct me to the point of no return. I'm hoping I can figure all this out in time, enough to be able to correct my own faulty way of living in survival mode. I'm not sure how to even start on getting on track, I have a few ideas but they are vague and may not even pan out.

If there's anything I have learned is that no one has it all figured out and everyone does their best with what they have and sometimes it doesn't work out as planned. And it's ok, just find a solution or a way back on track and keep moving forward. But whatever you do, if you can; don't get stuck in survival mode. Find some alternative, a friend, family member, co-worker, acquaintance, someone you still trust enough; to lean on for a moment to get yourself to a safe and secure environment. Don't let your own fear take the wheel and direct you in the story of your life. I promise you, it's not a great path forward. You can do better. You, dear reader, deserve better. Just try and don't give up. And for all those Enneagram sixes out there, keep the faith alive. It's just what you need to keep the fear in check, lean on your faith and use it as a tool not just for survival but to thrive. And, be happy. Be safe. Be ok. I know it can be easier

Because Trauma…

said than done, it seems much like a daily gamble if I'm going to take a risk of giving more faith or not.

Sally Taylor

Chapter Forty

It's not over yet.

It doesn't have to be.

Response: "I'm great with compartmentalization, I use it to get though difficult moments and continue going. I've done this for so long, if I'm not ready to talk; why push for me to address this when I've already moved on to keep going?"

Call it a skill related to my personality in personality theory or just call it a skill that I've learned to build up really well, either way; I can be really great with compartmentalizing. Maybe it's because of everything I've been through that it created an environment where I had to learn to be really good at it quickly, or maybe my own functioning was set up for this from the start. It's become just an automatic thing for me.

I know the past experiences contribute in some way. If it's something shocking enough where all you can do is get into the mindset of no emotion just function to get out of the situation, you've almost stripped yourself away into being almost robotic. In those moments, you'll hyper focus on getting out of the situation. All emotion takes a trunk ride as all logic takes the wheel. You think you're functioning but you're not, at least not properly.

Many may see it as being in a state of shock. That may be, but in this time you're less focused on the impact of the situation and how you feel about it and more focused on what it takes to get as far away from the situation as possible in the least amount of time. To do this, you compartmentalize. Set everything related to how you feel aside and the only relevant thing is creating a plan forward to getting out. In that moment, nothing else exists. There is no outside world to this situation, there's no other person who's going to be able to convince you to stop and tell them how you're feeling. The fact is, you're not. It's a defensive measure that some people take on to get through a difficult situation.

Sometimes compartmentalizing is a useful tool, sometimes it's excessive and a problem. If you compartmentalize just for a moment in a very traumatic time, like needing to flee from a very bad situation; you need all the focus on thinking rationally and it's helpful. There's also a right and a wrong way to go about it, and sometimes a fine line between the two. But you can't stay in that mindset for long, it really messes with a person. If you get so used to relying on compartmentalizing, then you've become excessive and will resort to it often, even when it's not necessary thus leading to more of a problem than a tool.

Because Trauma…

Someone who leads and has good management skills knows how to compartmentalize well. They have to for the job. In that respect, it's ok to get used to compartmentalizing. But when used as a tool for trauma response; it can become very unhealthy. A side effect to compartmentalizing too much in traumatic situations is you don't get the proper chance to process and let go of the emotions you've attached to the traumatic event. It becomes difficult for others to get through to you, you shut yourself off and don't let anyone in.

Not processing a traumatic event means you don't let yourself move past it and let it go. You don't heal, and instead let it continue to haunt you. I've spent years trying to find a way to compartmentalize and never have to deal with the past traumatic experiences. I was stubborn in refusing to talk about it and not wanting to focus on it at all. Trust me when I say, it doesn't work; especially when you are determined to work on bettering yourself to ultimately feel better and live better, you have to make it through that storm you've been outrunning.

Let it happen, process and allow yourself to let it all go. Probably the hardest decision is to finally let the storm catch up so you can process through it, because you know that's only the start and the rush of bad emotions will get worse. I'm sorry I don't have the best advice on getting through that, you just need the courage and determination and be very animate with yourself to not give up.

Believe fully that you are doing it to get to something so much better, because you are. Trust when I say it wouldn't be worth it if it wasn't hard. If it were so easy to overcome traumatic events there'd be nothing gained, nothing learned and nothing earned. You learn so much when overcoming traumatic events. You learn how to live better, how to deal with the situations better, how to feel better and how to be better. Your future matters and wouldn't it be worth a little time overcoming serious past traumatic events to really be able to thrive going forward?

I'm sorry to say the best advice I have is when you're ready, do what you can to process through it. Hang in there, don't give up, I believe in you and know you can do this. I'm very sorry that it came to battling a storm, it's truly difficult and my heart goes out to you.

Because Trauma…

Chapter Forty-One

Make your move,

take your stand.

Response: "I don't need pity, that's more hurtful than helpful. In the case of pity, just let me be. I'll take care of myself and the situation alone."

One thing that really frustrates me is when someone goes through a traumatic event and another person has pity on them. They just went through an extremely difficult situation and you've likely not been through it, why have pity? It's degrading and makes the person who went through the situation feel worse. Don't you think they feel bad enough?

If you've never been through a situation like that, you don't have to emphasize if you can't or don't want to. You can sympathize but please, don't pity. You might spark some hurt emotions from the individual who went through the traumatic situation and they just might lash out in a fit of anger.

The anger is from a "how dare you" mindset. Probably wanting to question why instead of helping or being kind is it necessary to pity or degrade. Pity means you feel sorry for someone, but not in a good way. It's almost like they are lower than you, status-wise or that they have done something wrong.

The truth is, if you somehow find yourself facing a traumatic event, it's not your fault and you don't need to have anyone else make you feel like it is in any way. I've had someone pity me before from a situation that caused me great distress. Yes, I lashed out, it hurt to have someone pity me instead of show empathy, sympathy or compassion.

I'm not great at communicating, especially when it's something I went through that was very traumatic; a medical professional looked down upon me with pity because I was upset over a traumatic situation and I wasn't communicating effectively. They took the situation wrong and instead of being kind they showed pity. It frustrated me so much. It was the first appointment with this medical professional as well as the last. I left knowing that I'd not return.

It wasn't worth going through the troubling event and then when you look to someone whose job it is to try to help you and instead, they just show pity; don't go back to that person, it truly isn't a good fit and not going to work out. For me, I was searching for a therapist, I found one I thought would be good but found out I couldn't go back and had to keep searching.

Pity makes someone feel worse than what they already feel. And if you're having pity on someone who experienced a traumatic event, you're testing their ability on not lashing out or worse, giving up and killing themselves. They're hurting and don't need to feel worse, showing pity will do just that and if they're already not in a great mindset; suicide is not off the table. Don't be someone who contributes their reasoning to commit suicide.

Because Trauma…

Sally Taylor

Reflection

Because Trauma…

Chapter Forty-Two

Find a way, to own

your hand. Lay all your cards...

Response: Some of my Personal Backstory...

I need to give backstory on a key core traumatic event I went through years ago. It's a past situation that I don't talk about to anyone now, though I have talked a little about it in the past to a handful of people. I stopped talking about it because I'm afraid to talk about it, I'm ashamed to bring it up, I haven't trusted anyone enough to share, and I'm afraid that if I do then I'd been seen differently. It's a part of my past I desperately wish I could forget ever existed. To act like it never happened and maybe one day it would fade out of existence and no longer be a part of my past. That's how much I've struggled with this. It's created some serious PTSD symptoms that still negatively affect me today. I'm bringing this up now, in this book because I need to stop seeing this as a part of my past I wish to forget ever existed and instead use it as this measurement of how much I've changed and improved since. Even though I'm dealing with serious PTSD symptoms from this, I've still made major improvement in other areas of my life, and that's something to be proud of and to celebrate, not to fear and try to erase from my own past.

I was in sixth grade. At the time, I couldn't make it through a day of school without escaping to the counselor's office or to hide in the bathroom. I hated school and hated home life. At home, I dealt with parents who didn't understand me and thought that ignoring me and beating me would be a solution. I'd leave that chaotic fear-filled environment to go to school where I was the prime target for being bullied. I struggled to make friends and when I did, they didn't last. Mainly because I was too fearful to trust them and would unintentionally sabotage the friendship because I couldn't give just a little trust in them. All the while I'm going through school each day in a full panic over bullies and having nowhere to turn for any help because the school took the side of the bullies instead of actually hearing what a very hurt and traumatized kid had to say. It really felt like the whole world was against me and not going to make better decisions to help a kid who lived in terror every minute of every day.

I had a full meltdown at school, I was eleven years old and in sixth grade. It was a matter of time by how things were going at home and school. My parents had to take me to get real medical help which landed me in a place that always said I spent time in a place that is hell residing, on earth. To understand the context of this statement, there needs to be a moment where you at least humor personality theory. I didn't know it at the time but that statement directly connects to an idea in personality theory. I've spent years now, researching personality theory and have reached depths of understanding that many don't have interest to go.

I'm not going to go too far into explaining personality theory because that would require writing another book, which some already have; I can give references on books and YouTube content creators who've really done well in explaining personality theory, at the end of this book. If any readers are interested in learning more.

I've researched my own personality and the way my mind works to try to understand myself better and what I found is the function that I lead with, would feel so destroyed if the person leading with that function were to spend time in prison. For my situation, I didn't spend time in prison but I spent time as an inpatient in the hospital mental wing. It may well have been prison because there didn't seem to be much difference.

For two weeks, I was told when to sleep, when to eat, when I had phone privileges, and when I could get some fresh air in a small fenced in courtyard. I spent the day watching videos that were meant to deter kids from doing drugs, all while not understanding why I was expected to take drugs. I was eleven years old and had very little understanding of two people engaging in sex, while a strange seventeen-year-old tried to hit on me and start a boyfriend/girlfriend relationship. I had nurses lie and manipulate me to get me to do what they wanted, participate in tests that I didn't agree to and didn't feel comfortable doing.

For two weeks, I lived in a place I called hell on earth; because that is what it was to me. It's affected me so greatly that I've developed PTSD symptoms from it. Every time I go to any hospital or medical building, my anxiety increases. It doesn't matter if I'm there visiting another person, I'm in full anxiety panic mode. Just a couple of years ago I was having a bad reaction to a medication and had to go to the emergency room. They admitted me and urged me to go on high blood pressure medication because my blood pressure was elevated too much.

I tried to tell them I didn't want to take the medication because I knew it was a symptom of PTSD from the time I spent in the hospital when I was eleven. They kept pressuring me and were trying to scare me into agreeing to take the medication by saying I could die from such high blood pressure, it worked and it was wrong. I spent a few days in the hospital before I was well enough to be discharged, the doctor gave me a script for blood pressure medication and again tried to pressure and scare me into agreeing to get it filled and take the medication.

I tried to explain that my blood pressure will go back down to normal once I'm out of the hospital and I tried to explain why but the doctor was too arrogant and unwilling to hear what I had to say. I felt like the doctor thought they knew everything and I was stupid to tell them anything medically related. Sure, you're a medical professional and you do know so much more of the medical field than what I do, but I've dealt with these PTSD symptoms for more than 18 years and I know what it's like and how it affects me.

I went home with the filled prescription and not even a day after called my mom telling her there was something wrong and I might have to go back to the emergency room. I couldn't do anything, and I could barely move without feeling dizzy or completely exhausted and off. What had happened was my blood pressure did drop back to normal, while I was taking medication for high blood pressure; which dropped my blood pressure to way below normal. My mom told me to stop taking the high blood pressure medication and to check in every once in a while, just to see if the issue would be resolved. Fifteen hours later I was back to feeling myself and able to function and get through the day without feeling dizzy, exhausted or off.

The concern with this doctor not caring enough to hear their patient they were trying to help is, I've struggled to trust long before ever meeting that doctor and my own trust in all medical professionals was hanging on a thin thread. This one medical professional's ability to be so arrogant in believing they knew everything and their patient wasn't worth hearing, has severely damaged all m trust I had in medical professionals. I'd rather risk it with a life-threatening illness than go to the doctor to get help. It's my PTSD symptoms on full control or having full say in the choices I make with any medical professionals now. It's a real problem, I know.

This moment in time, where I spent time in a hospital at eleven years old; plays a key role in many of the responses in this book. I'm too ashamed to bring it up, I don't trust anyone enough to talk about it, why should anyone care, it's my problem and I'll deal with it myself, I'm afraid to be seen differently, I'd rather forget and pretend it never existed to out-run the pain, and many more. This one moment in time has set up many more traumatic moments in my life, it led to being so drugged up I was like a living zombie, it's led my parents to believe that I'm too messed up to have anything to say that holds any value; I am seen as a broken unintelligent fool to my family and it hurts so much. They see me as incapable of holding real logical thought because I'm someone so messed up mentally and so emotional that it's impossible for anyone like that to have any sense of logic.

This one moment in time has affected my life in ways that it's going to take a lifetime to work on repairing. Even then, I'm not sure I can fix all the damage. There's likely real permanent brain damage from the massive amount of medications I had to take for so many years. I'm not trying to complain or lash out here, I'm just trying to give this information to hopefully reach this understanding of how serious the situation is and how much I've been affected by this traumatic event. It is what it is and I fully intend to spend what's left of my life repairing what damage I can and getting to something better.

Because Trauma…

Chapter Forty-Three

on the table.

If you need to…

Question: How do you heal from trauma?

There's no easy answer on how to heal from trauma. No one size fits all for therapy but it definitely helps. Finding the right therapist who can guide you through healing is important. But it's tough to find that right therapist for you. Sometimes you're going to one therapist after another, in search of someone who you feel you can connect with; it might take months, it might take years.

You have to want to work through it to actually get through it. If you're avoiding your own trauma and pent-up feelings from past traumas then working through them is not going to happen. It's going to have to be a conscious decision that you are determined and dedicated to. You have to really want it. If you don't, the passion and drive to get to something better won't be there; the intent won't be there, so you'll continue to live with the pain and past trauma.

Because Trauma…

You almost have to be so annoyed with yourself for taking the route of avoiding, that you finally say, "Bring it on, I want to tackle that storm," and actually grit through it. It won't be fun; it won't be easy. It's going to seem like hell and you're going to experience so much more pain. Some days it will be to the point of unbearable. Where you're unsure if you'll even survive or have a future. Don't listen to that voice in your head. You will, you just got to work through the storm to get to the other side. You'll see, it does get better.

It's like it takes the absolute worst point of your life, your lowest point, rock bottom; before you can work your way back out of the hole, towards something better. I'm sorry to say, but sometimes that's what it takes. It's not fun, it's not pleasant; it's very much like your own hell. I'm sorry, now get to work on digging your way out. You can do it, I know it. Because I have. I'm not completely out but I've made such significant progress. That's how it's going to be, and I have every intent to keep digging my way out.

In some ways, I think that's the point to life; to keep working on self-improvement and digging your way out of your own hell on earth. It shapes people into something greater. And if you have the pleasure of experiencing trauma early in life, well; you've got a head start. No, it's not a great way of looking at it but humor this perspective for a moment; someone who's not been through truly difficult situations won't have the knowledge or real experience in getting themselves out.

If they were to have such difficulty later in life, it's going to be quite a hit that might be more of a challenge to dig out of at that stage in life. I'm not saying start out going through the most hellish experiences to forge your own defenses and skills at tackling the worst, I'm saying see your own difficulties as key learning experiences that you just might be ahead of the game at. See the best in the worst situations because that's the best way to get through them.

Don't let anyone make you feel impotent or weak for the trauma's you've endured. Don't let anyone put you down for them or pity you. You don't need their pity; you need empathy or sympathy. You are not weak for struggling through such a difficult situation. You've just run into a challenge, face to face, that is going to take much learning and growth from you.

And that's a beautiful thing to be able to learn something great. Some great way of overcoming some difficult situation. Sure, in the moment you won't see it that way. That's fine, it's natural. That's why empathy or sympathy is important. Because you're in a situation that hurts and you don't need harsh critics tearing you down more, you need kindness, compassion and maybe a little guidance and some people cheering you on. You need someone in your corner rooting for you saying they have your back and will support you if you need it.

You are not weak, you are forging tools, skills, to be strong enough to overcome and be better. Think of it that way. It will be tough in the moment, I get it. I don't always approach a traumatic situation excited to forge a new skill. In fact, I never have before but rather go unhinged until I find that key learning opportunity.

It hurts and there's a lot of pain from it. It's very difficult to see the silver lining in these moments but with practice, you'll start to see it sooner. And working to something better moves much smoother. Doesn't mean there's less pain, I truly wish there was; but you'd be able to bear more and get through it quicker.

If you do have someone in your life that shows pity first and would contribute more trauma and pain to an already difficult situation, then I'm sorry to say that maybe they don't have the best interest at heart for you. Do you really need them in your life? If you say yes, stop yourself and really think. Why? What positivity are they bringing to the relationship?

Is there a financial reason? Then find another way around the problem to get distance from them. Are you married to them? Then maybe separation or divorce is a better solution. You say you love them; I get that, but do you think they truly love you or are they just saying they do for a means to their end. An ulterior motive.

Whatever your reason, it's valid but yet, it's not. You're scared and lying to yourself. Trust me, I know; I'm a professional at being afraid and lying to myself. I had such limiting beliefs on what I could do or what situation I had to stay in because I had such little confidence in myself. I believed I'd fail at getting to something better or that something better didn't exist.

Understand that lying to yourself is a defense mechanism you use in an attempt to protect yourself from the unknown, which at times can be far scarier than the actual traumatic situations you've endured. Here's the trick, knowing not to listen to that and going for something better anyways. Even if you might not see that light at the end of the tunnel, that doesn't mean it's not there. There just may be an obstacle blocking it or maybe you are too far away to see it. Take that leap of faith and save yourself, get to a better life.

If that means cutting ties with someone who doesn't have good intentions or the best interest at heart, then I'm sorry that's what it's going to take. It won't be fun; it will be terrifying. But you go for it anyways, give yourself a fighting chance, metaphorically speaking. Take the steps you need to work on what you need for a better life. A happier life. You deserve it. Remember that and believe it because some days it will be hard to believe.

Don't blame yourself, whatever the traumatic event; it's not your fault. A common situation children go through when parents' divorce is blaming themselves for their parents' separation. They believe that if they had been a better kid or done something better, it would have saved their parents' marriage. Truth is, no part of the decision of the parents to divorce is in any way the kids' fault. The same goes for any traumatic experience. No one asks to go through a situation that traumatizes them, no one asks to experience real pain; it happens and it's very unpleasant. It's not the fault of the individual going through the situation, don't think it is and don't listen to anyone who says it is. If you are blaming yourself, forgive yourself; and allow yourself to finally heal. It is not your fault.

Going through a traumatic experience can really affect a person's self-esteem and self-worth. I've struggled with feeling like I wasn't good enough or didn't matter as much as the next person, much more than I'd like to admit. Truth is, I've been there too much and it's not true. If you're going through these feelings of others are better, don't let that thought pattern win, it's wrong; you matter just as much as the next person.

Think of it this way, you've been through a difficult situation, I'm sorry but instead of falling into the trap of self-hatred and thinking everyone is more deserving or better than you, learn to use that set back as a useful tool, a way you can refine and help others in the future. That, I guarantee is very valuable and much needed. Sure, it's not great that it takes a traumatic situation, but instead of letting this trouble win and defeat you; why not conquer it and forge it into something much better?

You are also not alone in this, there are many other individuals in that same defeated feeling thinking everyone is much better than them, even thinking you are better than them. You see, it's all perspective; a perspective that's not helpful and is not set in stone, you can change it and you can come out of this ok. Sure, you're not really interested in hearing this when you're so hurt and defeated by the traumatic event; I've been there before and I don't appreciate anyone telling me to "look at the bright side."

It's not helpful in that moment, in that moment you need support and a chance to recover, heal. But once the charged emotions of the situation passes and you're able to see your situation more clearly, that's when this message will be helpful. Just don't give in to the defeat before you have that chance to process and heal enough to think more clearly. You matter and you are so needed for this world, just as much as your neighbor.

I can't tell you how many times I've gotten advice from medical professionals or people that care about me and I've wanted to shove it back in their face telling them they're not helpful. I struggled to believe that there'd be a day that the advice would be helpful. It takes time but I assure you, that time will come and you'll be able to jump into action on making changes for a better life. But the struggle through the difficult situation may only be the start of the battle, some things are quite difficult to change; especially when it's how you've grown up and lived every day of your life.

The real challenge is breaking those habits to set your sights on something better, a different lifestyle or something can be difficult to change. It takes motivation, dedication and time; but trust me, it's worth it. You might not see it until weeks, months or years after; when your life has significantly changed for the better. Do your best, you will get through this, this isn't a science; it's an art. There is no one right way, you just have to try.

Sally Taylor

Chapter Forty-Four

Take your chance,

to grit through it...

Final Examples and Closing Thoughts...

One of the scariest and most difficult things to hear from a medical professional, more specifically a psychiatrist or therapist is them asking in wonder how the person seeing them has not committed suicide yet. Like it's an unusual thing and this person should have ended their lives by now. I've been through that a few times. It twists my thoughts and feelings up in nots and I don't understand how that could be a question and, I struggle to respond.

I'm sure from my history, a good number of different versions of this question could be asked, why am I not an alcoholic, why haven't I turned to illegal drugs, and so on. Truth is, I don't have a great answer for this. I can see now all the times I wish I was in that dedicated mindset of ending my life. Something always pulls me away from that ledge at the last moment. Maybe it's my own internal drive to keep going, maybe my stubbornness to not let these traumatic experiences win, maybe my optimism keeps me from making that final move. Maybe, I've defied the odds so much that it's now a game to keep defying odds and getting that close to the edge just to pull myself back. Or maybe, it has something to do with just an act of God.

I don't have a great answer because I don't understand it myself. I know that's a terrible answer and the concern from that is there's no good answer keeping me from making those life ending decisions. I get that, all I can say is I've had so many times where it would have made sense to be that fed up and done but, here I am; writing this book.

I've been through my fair share of therapists. I spent the few years searching for a right fit or match and I found one that I stayed with for around ten years. It took every bit of eight for this therapist to get me to open up and it wasn't so much my therapist's accomplishment but my poetry professor. Then came the time when I was driven to figure myself out and work on getting myself to something better. I dove into many outlets like interest in the paranormal, interest in journalism, and media production.

I found a path with the paranormal that I needed to explore in-depth, and that's when I ran into difficulties with this therapist. I found myself filtering what I said because I knew it went against what this therapist believed in. That's not how therapy works and I knew it. I tried opening up a little on my search through all things paranormal and it didn't go well, with my therapist's religious beliefs; she felt the need to speak up on her personal opinion on the paranormal, as not real and should not be looked into. Then decided to get even more religious on me.

At the time, I didn't believe in any religion. I was borderline accepting that I was an atheist because I couldn't find a religious belief to commit to. I tended to stray away from any conversation that had a focus on religion or politics because I knew I wouldn't convince anyone to believe in what I believed and no one could change my mind in what to believe in. I've been through enough conversations to know that if you disagree on religious beliefs, others tend to jump at the chance to try to convert you. It's not being respectful of the person, who may already have their own valid beliefs and it's forcing yours onto them; which is a situation that no one would enjoy experiencing. I had no intention on forcing my beliefs onto another, I didn't understand why someone else couldn't have the same respect for me.

That's what I ran into with this therapist and I knew it was time to make a change to a new therapist. After ten years, I wasn't too eager to begin that long search to find another good fit, but I knew if I wanted to work on healing and getting better; I needed the guidance from a therapist I could feel comfortable opening up to.

I found another therapist and settled in with being prepared to really open up. All the therapists in the past have been pretty straight forward and I was walking into this new option with the same expectations. That's when I realized the challenge with this therapist. None of my previous therapists had broken out in tears over my story and it worked for me because if someone's getting too emotional around me, whether they show it or not; I'm like a sponge for emotions, I will pick up on that so quickly. I'm already broken up over my situation and having a therapist cry too is like getting a double dose of troubling emotions. I wasn't prepared for that and it caught me off guard.

To this day, I haven't said anything about it. But it still affects me every time. I wonder, during those moments; how can someone now be crying over my story? I've been through so much and it's taken such a toll for so long, how can someone now be feeling for me. After everything, now someone feels for me. It's a little late for that, isn't it? I've already gone through so much and not interested in someone babying me in emotions by crying over my story.

It's not a great train of thought, but it happens. I'm so used to having my own emotions trampled over and no one really caring enough to genuinely feel for me like that; I'm unsure of how to deal with it. It really messes with me to have someone feel for me like that instead of not caring too much, disregarding, or trampling my emotions. My thoughts spin and I'm stuck with this unsettling feeling of how do I deal with this or how do I be ok with this? Really the best thing I know to do is to say nothing because I'm afraid if I do, I'd be disrespectful to their emotions from my own confusion; and that's not something I want to do.

The circumstances have changed for me now; and they can change for you, dear reader. Yes, I'm still seeing the therapist that cries over my story, and I still haven't said anything. I've found my drive, my reason to keep going. No, I'm not out of the woods of trauma yet, but I'm doing everything I can to work my way out and to a better future. Life is still very painful and depressing but I do see that light at the end of this very dark tunnel. I see the progress I've made and I can see the future where it gets better. It's worth fighting for, it's worth hanging around to get to something better.

I reached that point of being truly fed up and done with my situation and reached the understanding that I'd be the one that would have to do something to get myself out. I guess it truly does take reaching rock bottom to finally be able to pull yourself up and work towards something better. It seems like my situation here. The down side is being at your lowest, but the good thing is once you are there; there's only one way left to go. Mainly because you know you're at rock bottom and are still alive, so why not try something different; try for something better.

It's a long haul that takes everything in you to keep going but have faith that your own instincts will help guide you through. In this case, be stubborn and don't allow yourself to give up. No matter how annoying it gets, forge stubbornness into resilience and give yourself that fighting chance for something better. Trust me, it can be done; because I have.

Because Trauma…

Chapter Forty-Five

Find that drive, for your better future. …You're worth it…

What this all means…?

I wish I had a great answer for the medical professionals, who had asked such challenging questions of how I hadn't committed suicide yet. I know how concerning not having an answer is. To not have an answer to that question is concerning because it sparks the question as to what is keeping me from making that choice?

Best answers I have are, I'm resilient and stubborn. I don't give up easily no matter how much I'd like to at times. I can look back at my life and see so many times where I've defied some outlandish odds, where so many didn't think possible. I still deal with those situations to this day, and they have yet to stop me.

The most current situation, at the end of this fall 2021 semester, I will graduate with a Bachelor's Degree. Because of what high school I attended for over three years, it's rare for a student from there to get an Associate's Degree. Sure, it took a little more time because I was not interested in school, but I defied the odds and now have an Associate's Degree. By December of 2021, I'll have a Bachelor's Degree. If getting an Associate's Degree is rare, then getting a Bachelor's Degree must be unheard of, right? Yet, here I am, about to defy another outlandish odd.

Sure, the comments of how unusual it is for me to have an Associate's Degree has taken quite a toll on me, it's worse for my Bachelor's but it hasn't deterred me. I'm still putting my best effort in classes to get another step closer to graduation. I am very stubborn, when I set my mind on something; like a goal, I go for it and refuse to give up. The same can be said for traumatic situations and situations where everyone else doesn't see how I've managed to keep going, I had some drive where I couldn't allow myself to give up. Even in those many times where I wish I would give up. Those troubling and dark days where I saw no end to the emotional pain other than escaping the only real way I knew of, an ultimate end.

I think it also took finding a new relationship with depression, anxiety and fear. Before, I'd struggle to find a sense of peace, an escape from the anxiety and depression. But after so many attempts and all of which were fails, and feeling so defeated by this; I decided to change my own understanding and perspective on depression and anxiety. I decided to accept it as a real part of who I am and instead of drowning from it, work with it to find a good balance of taking care of my everyday needs and my emotional needs all while knowing the depression and anxiety will get better but wouldn't ever go away, it's forever a part of my life.

Speaking of fear, that's something I'm still unsure on how to overcome or even work with. I've lived in this mindset of survival mode for so long; it's really all I know. That mindset is pure fear based. While being stuck in survival mode, I'm always looking for the next threat or concerning situation; trying to dodge completely or buffer the impact as much as I possibly can. Trust runs scarce because I don't trust my own judgement on who I can trust. So, instead, I learn to rely solely on trusting myself knowing full well I can't even do that. I doubt myself every day, question my own logic and tear it apart to make sure I'm right.

The unique relationship I have with fear is no picnic. I wrestle every day with my own frustration over allowing fear to have such power. I say I'll do better today and not let fear call the shots but do I ever really do that? If I'm being realistic, I don't know how to make any decision that is not fear based or factors in the aspect of fear. I don't think I'm capable of that, at least not yet. So, I don't do better, I still am tripped up by my own fear calling the shots. And I don't know how to work with that. I don't even know if it's possible. Can you use fear as an advantage rather than let it call the shots? Is it possible to have a good working relationship with fear? Even when it's fear that's based out of pure survival mode, the fear you've lived with your entire life as you navigated this world feeling so underprepared and unsafe?

Instead of seeing depression and anxiety as my enemy, I chose to start seeing them as troubled family members that you just always have around. Sure, a very strange metaphor for this but the point is not to fight against the depression and anxiety but to find a middle ground where you can work around it or have it in your life but not take power over you. Acknowledge it but don't let it drive you. Respect it and accept that it's probably always going to be around. Sounds bizarre, I know; but it works. It lines up with giving yourself permission to not be ok, and have more compassion for yourself; giving yourself the chance to heal on the terms that maybe you don't want but truly need. Because this does take time, and I get it; that's not always ideal. It's necessary.

If it helps to find a belief system to cling onto, do that. I've been very difficult and even stubborn in believing in something when it comes to religion. If it helps to go on late night rant drives where you drive for an hour or so crying and screaming at your steering wheel, do that; just in a way that doesn't cause an accident. If it helps to just go outside and run until you tire yourself out, do that. If it helps to journal, do that. If it helps to write a book, do that. Find your own method of processing and coping and, if you have to, cling to it. Use it to your advantage.

Don't fall into the trap of suffering alone, that doesn't work out well. Find someone you trust to talk to, actually open up and get real with them. Be ok with not being ok and have faith that the person you trust enough to open up to will understand and respect that. Find your voice and don't be afraid to use it, sing. If that means literal for you, great; or it might just mean speaking up about your situation. Be someone who can spark change for other's to not fall into the same troubling situations, if that's what it takes.

Turn your hellish situation into a learning experience and a path forward to helping others, but only when you truly know you're ready and capable of being that spark of change. Give it time, you'll know when you're ready and can handle it. Be patient with yourself. Healing takes time and the readiness to heal, find peace and be done with past traumas. You can tell yourself you're done and ready but you won't truly be until you start taking action on getting to something better and you have that drive where you know you'll get there and you won't give up.

Don't let the genuine curiosity of medical professionals, or anyone around you, defeat you by asking such questions like how you haven't committed suicide yet. The point is you haven't, you're still here and that's something to celebrate. The questions and curiosity really don't matter, your own wellbeing is what matters. If it bothers you, challenge them by asking why they'd ask such a thing. Stand your ground and take care of yourself. You are worth it, you matter; it's so great you're here, alive.

If a medical professional tears up over your story, maybe that's infinitive to use it in the future as a motivational speech. Speak up, spark change, help others. When you get to the point of helping another, it has the same effect of helping you too; you still heal from your past when you get a chance to make a positive change for someone else in their life. It doesn't make the situation from your past ok, or even a good reason to go through it; you're just using your past situation as an advantage to help another and continue to heal yourself.

It's not easy going through a traumatic experience, it typically pushes you into a fight, flight, or freeze response and can spark a range of negative emotions that long outlast the actual event. Coping or healing from the traumatic situation is another story, some might say it's much more difficult than the actual traumatic event; because for some people it's like the event hadn't ended and they keep reliving the horrific or troubling moment over, many times on a daily basis. Breaking yourself out of that mindset to allow yourself to heal is no easy feat.

For some people it might take getting to their absolute worst in order to have only one way left to go, other's it might take assistance or support from people around that care and want what's best for the individual that's still wrestling with the traumatic experience, and some may just need a little time and space to process and find their best path and may already have great coping mechanisms. Not everyone needs help after a difficult and traumatic situation, some may already have the understanding and tools to process and cope. It just takes knowing yourself, how you work and what you need. Stay true to yourself and take care of yourself, if you need assistance; don't be afraid to ask.

Because Trauma…

Sally Taylor

<u>Because Trauma</u>

Heart beating faster, now
pain ruling your fear, now
train of thought derailing, now
you can't see past the pain, now

>a glimmer of hope, so fleeting.
>Heart heavy, eyes steady,
>and wide.
>You pray for that moment
>of peace.

Pause. Wait. Not here, not now.
Panic.
Another round of hurt,
another round of screaming

in your own head.
You hope that instead,
you find someone not red.

>With hate.
>With anger.
>With rage.
>They don't see you as you, now.

Because Trauma...

    Their anger everlasting.
    Long after the event's passing.
    A reoccurring nightmare, for you.
    A faded memory, in their journey.
    Their fear leading their way.

They are lost, misguided,
into thinking, their action
was a reaction, justified.
Not cruel, not heartless.

Being hateful, creating
mass destruction in your
own mind. Deconstruction.

    The very fabric of your
    wellbeing, your self-esteem.
    Don't fall for it. Never easy,
    don't listen to your own mind,

        Your own train of thought, sabotaging.
        Don't listen to your own defeating,
        self-talk, of all the...
        Not worth it's,
        and I deserve it's—Say you're fine,

when you know you're not.

Sally Taylor

    It's simple, here,
    put on a facade.
    Say you're ok.

Hide it. Fight it.
Ignore it. Bury it.
Conceal it. Heal it.

    You know you can't.
    That's not how this works,
    it's haunting…how your past,
    always finds a way,

        to find you, hunt you,
        catch up to you, blind you,
        keep you guessing,
        panicking,
        fearful.

    Will you ever be whole?
  Will you ever make it
    out of this…
    dark tunnel of life.

With no light to guide,
and no guide to light,
your way through this

Because Trauma…

    seemingly ever endless
    darkness.
    It's defining.
    Pulling you, down, down,

        deeper. Into this abyss.
        Struggling to breathe,
        there's one way,
        swim harder,
        for that surface,

    keep fighting…
    …for your purpose.
    You still have a chance,
    It's not over yet.

It doesn't have to be.
Make your move,
take your stand.

    Find a way, to own
    your hand. Lay all your cards…
    on the table.
    If you need to…

        Take your chance,
        to grit through it…
        Find that drive, for your

better future.
...You're worth it...

Because Trauma…

References

For further reading:

Disclaimer – There are many more books on enneagram and personality theory, these books are just the key top two that I've used that has helped in my understanding.

Beatrice Chestnut (2013). The Complete Enneagram: 27 Paths to Greater Self-Knowledge. She Writes Press. https://www.amazon.com/Complete-Enneagram-Paths-Greater-Self-Knowledge/dp/1938314549/ref=sr_1_16?crid=W9NGQ4VUP8X7&dchild=1&keywords=ennegram&qid=1634771886&s=books&sr=1-16

Joel Mark Witt and Antonia Dodge (2018). Personality Hacker: Harness the Power of Your Personality Type to Transform Your Work, Relationships, and Life. Ulysses Press. https://www.amazon.com/Personality-Hacker-Harness-Transform-Relationships/dp/1612437664/ref=sr_1_1?dchild=1&keywords=personality+hacker&qid=1634772250&s=books&sr=1-1

YouTube Content Creators:

Because Trauma...

Disclaimer – These are content creators I've followed and have learned from, there are many more great content creators on YouTube that have a nice developed understanding of the material, these are not the only two; just the two I've followed for years, and found their content understandable and very insightful.

Objective Personality (2010)
C.S. Joseph (2017)

Final Thoughts...

My fear after completing this book is not of all my experiences finally out to the world but fear of this book defining me. I don't want to be remembered by this book and the experiences I've been through, the amount of understanding I have of traumatic experiences or even the fact that I've overcome traumatic experiences. Instead, I just wish to be seen as just another person. I know that the expectation in that is unrealistic because I did create this book and this is my hard work diving into the most difficult moments of my past to attempt to make something good from it. And if this does end up helping someone in their own life, even just one person; I can't help but to appreciate this book for that opportunity and see this as a necessity and not something to worry about being remembered by. Still, I am human and sometimes I have unrealistic worries or fears. I'll eventually get over it.

~ ~ ~

Afterwards

One last focus for this book, and I'm starting to understand the importance and it's likely the most important in this entire book. It's something I've struggled to grasp my entire life up until very recently. It's a concept I'm horrible with but looking to improve. Taking a very personal move here, I must include this in my book:

To the people in my life that's greatly affected me in such a negative way, with all the traumatic situations; I know I've not responded well. I know I've made many mistakes in the process of trying to avoid or work through them, my approach has been wrong from the start. And that may be all because I've refused to find a way to forgive. I didn't see how I could because I've been hurt and didn't want to forgive someone who kept dishing out more difficult and even abusive situations. I was so very wrong in this.

Because Trauma...

I wrote this book because I needed to, it was my way of processing through everything. I wrote this book in hopes that it could be helpful to someone who may need it. I wrote it with the little hope that I'd be proven wrong by what I wrote in this book, and I'd actually be heard and understood; that maybe things can change for the better in the family dynamic. That's a hope I'll hold onto but understand that it may not work out. And it's fine. This book is intended to help someone, if that be helping medical professionals understand a little better, then great; or if it helps someone in such a mess of a situation that just needs a little encouragement.

A short time ago, a member in my small group commented and recommended a book to read to everyone in the group, I was interested and bought a copy of the book to read. The book is by John W. Nieder and Thomas M. Thompson titled Forgive and Love Again. It is now a book I highly recommend if you or someone you know is struggling to forgive.

Hands down, one of the best books I could have ever read in my life; I'm so grateful that this group member suggested it. I will be returning to our regularly scheduled group meet next time leading with the most heartfelt thank you for this group member.

It opened my eyes to understanding forgiveness in a way I never saw before and I now can see how possible and imperative it is to reach forgiveness. I'm not completely through reading the book, still only being in chapter seven; I've got much more to read but if the first six chapters has this much impact, I'm eager to keep reading.

Now the most important part of my book, I know I haven't approached situations in the past in the best way, I know I've reacted out of hurt and refused to forgive for many, many years. I know I was wrong in refusing to forgive and it's shaped how I am today in dramatic ways, those of which are not good. I know I've got a long way to go on moving past my past but I see the key now as finding forgiveness. It's not going to be an easy statement solution and all is right and good, it's going to take many times of me repeating to myself and God that I forgive. It's going to be a repeated mantra until I fully feel and believe it and I've found my way to forgiving.

This is my forgiveness promise:

To everyone I've refused to forgive over the years because I couldn't allow myself to forgive despite the emotional and sometimes physical pain, I am making this conscious decision now, that's long overdue; I'm sorry for not forgiving you when I needed to and it really was the best and just thing to do, I understand and am making this conscious decision now to say, it may take repeated mantras but I do forgive you. I forgive friends who emotionally and physically hurt, they didn't know the impact or hurt they were acting out. I forgive family for any form of hurt, I didn't contribute anything good by refusing to forgive and it wasn't ok of me. It's going to take time, repeating a mantra of forgiveness, but I forgive over everything I've held onto over the years.

Even so, I forgive you, doesn't always mean I'm able to return to the same toxic environment. It wouldn't be right for anyone if I did. I'm still focused on finding my true path towards my future, building bridges and boundaries when needed; I forgive the actions of all the wrong, but I'm not willing to go back to that same environment. I hold nothing to those people in my past, I release all resentment, anger, hurt, and pain from past interactions. But I know it's not wise to return to those situations and individuals. I wish everyone from my past the very best in their lives, hope all is well and they too find their way to moving past the past, if they haven't yet.

...I forgive you.

Mom,

I know it's been rough for the both of us. I know I've lashed back in ways I shouldn't have. The past six months has seemed like I didn't exist. I disappeared to figure everything out. Yes, I debated on staying forever gone. Out of respect for what this book publication has led to, I'm reaching out finally, after six months of trying to figure things out. I've progressed closer to graduation, I've published a book and now that book, this book is gaining traction. I've gone to interviews for possible job opportunities, attended a few events on-campus for honors cords for graduation. I've excelled at the church internship. They've become like a family to me. It's going to be hard to leave if there becomes a situation, to leave for the job. I've been lowered and now off of all the medications that I've taken for so many years, it's been a while now and I've figured out what it's like to not take so many medications. My doctors are baffled and proud. But it's still a challenge. I know I'm still trying to get to some normalcy without the medications. I've missed family, everyone really. But I couldn't worry about family and work on where I needed to be. I'm not mad, I'm not angry, I just want to move past all of it. That's what publishing has given me, my chance to move past it all. I'd love to be a part of the family again, but I know I can't walk back to how things were. It's not right for me or anyone else in the family. Things need to change, I don't expect all at once and very dramatically, it's going to take time; I know this. But, for there to be a good family dynamic and future, we need to work together towards getting to something better. I know you're very hesitant on making changes, but I really need your support on this. We need to work on getting to something better, together. That's the best way it will work and that's the best way we can have a working family relationship going forward.

I know I'll be cautious; I've been hurt too much not to be, I'm trying but living feeling unsafe and feeling disregarded has some lasting damage. I do love you, I always will; you're my mom, I'm incapable of not loving you. I still don't trust you, I'm not sure how I could; the games of saying one thing but doing another has really pushed past my ability to trust. I'm sorry for the direction that everything has taken, I needed some time and I'm hoping we can now work on something better. This book is such an accomplishment and yes, there's stuff that's going to hurt. It hasn't been easy for me to publish this, but I needed this. I had to find a way to get past it, since I felt like I was dealing with it alone, this was my best option. I'm hoping you can understand that when I was writing, I was in the middle of this mess. Now, months later, I've worked past much of it and am hoping to rebuild a good future with family. It won't be the same relationship as before, I'm still cautious to trust; I'm still hurting and going to prioritize my safety, protection and wellbeing.

~~~ END ~~~

Because Trauma…

www.ingramcontent.com/pod-product-compliance
Lightning Source LLC
Chambersburg PA
CBHW052308220526
45472CB00001B/31